AF768174

ENDOCRINOLOGY RESEARCH AND CLINICAL DEVELOPMENTS

QUALITY OF LIFE IN ENDOCRINE DISEASES

ENDOCRINOLOGY RESEARCH AND CLINICAL DEVELOPMENTS

Additional books in this series can be found on Nova's website under the Series tab.

Additional e-books in this series can be found on Nova's website under the e-book tab.

ENDOCRINOLOGY RESEARCH AND CLINICAL DEVELOPMENTS

QUALITY OF LIFE IN ENDOCRINE DISEASES

ERIKA CESAR DE OLIVEIRA NALIATO
EDITOR

NOVA BIOMEDICAL

New York

Copyright © 2015 by Nova Science Publishers, Inc.

All rights reserved. No part of this book may be reproduced, stored in a retrieval system or transmitted in any form or by any means: electronic, electrostatic, magnetic, tape, mechanical photocopying, recording or otherwise without the written permission of the Publisher.

For permission to use material from this book please contact us:
nova.main@novapublishers.com

NOTICE TO THE READER

The Publisher has taken reasonable care in the preparation of this book, but makes no expressed or implied warranty of any kind and assumes no responsibility for any errors or omissions. No liability is assumed for incidental or consequential damages in connection with or arising out of information contained in this book. The Publisher shall not be liable for any special, consequential, or exemplary damages resulting, in whole or in part, from the readers' use of, or reliance upon, this material. Any parts of this book based on government reports are so indicated and copyright is claimed for those parts to the extent applicable to compilations of such works.

Independent verification should be sought for any data, advice or recommendations contained in this book. In addition, no responsibility is assumed by the publisher for any injury and/or damage to persons or property arising from any methods, products, instructions, ideas or otherwise contained in this publication.

This publication is designed to provide accurate and authoritative information with regard to the subject matter covered herein. It is sold with the clear understanding that the Publisher is not engaged in rendering legal or any other professional services. If legal or any other expert assistance is required, the services of a competent person should be sought. FROM A DECLARATION OF PARTICIPANTS JOINTLY ADOPTED BY A COMMITTEE OF THE AMERICAN BAR ASSOCIATION AND A COMMITTEE OF PUBLISHERS.

Additional color graphics may be available in the e-book version of this book.

Library of Congress Cataloging-in-Publication Data

ISBN: 978-1-63463-911-8
Library of Congress Control Number: 2014959999

Published by Nova Science Publishers, Inc. † New York

Contents

Preface

Having been working in the field of Endocrinology for 15 years, it is easy to observe the wide clinical variety of the different Endocrine diseases. After some time, it becomes obvious that this spectrum involves more than biochemical variations.

My mentors, Dr. Annamaria Colao and Dr. Alice Violante, introduced me to the concept of "Quality of life" when I was working on my PhD thesis and we began to study this aspect in patients with prolactinoma. However, to the best of our knowledge, until this moment there is no collection in the literature particularly dedicated to analyze the effects of the various Endocrine diseases on quality of life.

This collection contains an extensive review on data published in the literature regarding quality of life in different Endocrine diseases. The first chapter intends to familiarize the reader with the concept of quality of life. In addition, each of the following chapters was structured in order to provide a quick review on the main aspects of an Endocrine disease and its consequences on quality of life. In the second chapter, the authors discuss the aspects of quality of life in non-functioning pituitary tumors. Another frequent type of pituitary tumor, the prolactinoma, is the object of Chapter 3. The quality of life of patients with acromegaly and growth hormone deficiency is the theme of the fourth chapter, and that of subjects with Cushing's syndrome is the focus of Chapter 5. Hypogonadism in men and women and its consequences to quality of life are discussed in Chapter 6, while quality of life of patients with hypo- and hyperthyroidism is analyzed in Chapter 7. Finally, Diabetes Mellitus and Obesity and their consequences on quality of life are discussed, respectively, in Chapters 8 and 9.

The authors hope that this collection can help our readers to improve their understanding of this fascinating aspect of the Endocrine diseases.

Erika C. O. Naliato

In: Quality of Life in Endocrine Diseases ISBN: 978-1-63463-911-8
Editor: Erika Cesar de Oliveira Naliato © 2015 Nova Science Publishers, Inc.

Chapter 1

Introduction: Quality of Life

Antonio C. M. Costa Junior, Elza F. S. Cerqueira and Erika C. O. Naliato*

Center of Studies Ricardo A T Castilho of the Teresópolis Medical Association, Brazil

Keywords: Quality of life, endocrine diseases

The sense of well-being and quality of life (QoL) is fomented throughout the whole human development. According to Victor et al. (2000) [1], QoL includes an ample spectrum of areas. QoL models extend from the satisfaction with life or social well-being to those based on concepts of independence, control, social competence and cognition. According to the World Health Organization (WHO), the expression "quality of life" was used for the first time by Lyndon Johnson, former president of the United States of America, in the beginning of his term to declare that it would be the most important priority of his government. Smith (2001) [2] considers that the concept of well-being has changed since the middle of the XX century. Until then, it signified only the disposition of material means (food, housing, access to health services, social actions, and financial security). Nowadays, it also relates to less tangible dimensions (sense of security, personal dignity, means of reaching personal goals, satisfaction with life, happiness, and self-esteem).

* Correspondence to: erikanaliato@uol.com.br

The notion of QoL has been altered and encompasses resources and the right to seize life. Nevertheless, its concept is not unanimous. Campbell (1981) [3] considered that satisfaction and happiness are different concepts; satisfaction implicates in judgment or cognitive experience, while happiness suggests an affective experience. Recently, there has been a consensus that satisfaction is part of QoL. Campbell [3] showed that the subjects spoke of satisfaction when inquired about QoL. Other studies that have been evaluating QoL in every age group, since 1965, demonstrated that satisfaction and well-being were important subjective factors for QoL. The progressive improvement in certain indicators of daily life, such as education, income, health, and type of occupation, should affect life satisfaction positively, but QoL seems to have diminished. This seeming contradiction may be the result of variations of importance attributed to the above mentioned indicators. QoL is, therefore, a concept that encompasses a wide range of human experiences. In the medical area, it is related to the effects of a disease in a patient, corresponding to the health-related QoL, and stands the focus of studies that evaluate QoL in patients with certain diseases [4].

The Evaluation of Quality of Life

The QoL of a certain patient is a complex category that comprehends cultural, economic, and educational aspects of the studied subject. Consequently, QoL evaluation is problematic, considering its subjective aspect [5-8]. The attempt to evaluate QoL appeared parallel to the first definition of health, in 1946. Since then, aspects related with patients' health have predominated. Then, several methodological tools have been developed in order to evaluate QoL. Table 1 presents some tools used in this evaluation [5-8].

Table 1. Methods to evaluate Quality of life

Action State
APACHE pontuation system
QoL indexes (Karnofsky Scale)
Self-evaluation scale
QoL Questionnaires
Individual interviews
Focus groups

Any of the above mentioned tools can be used in different levels [5-8]:

- Individual: evaluation of QoL in each individual.
- Group: evaluation of QoL in a group of patients or subjects.
- Population: evaluation of QoL in a group of population of patients with specific diseases, in order to assess the disease or its treatment.

Currently, studies on QoL are based on questionnaires, the most frequently used research method. There are multiple questionnaires available at “ProQolid”, a data bank of psychometric tools. This bank comprehends tools that can qualify QoL, divided according to the research focus – general tools (used in healthy populations and patients), disease-specific tools, and population-specific tools [5-8].

The WHO’s models of QoL, as well as its questionnaires, are worldly recognized for their complexities and practicality. WHO describes QoL as a very heterogeneous, specific, individual, and sophisticated category [5-8].

Besides the present QoL, hypothetic QoL in the absence of disease can also be evaluated. For the latter, in general, one aspect of the life of the patient is related to the hypotheses – e.g., “How would your diet be, if you did not have diabetes?” [5-8].

QoL-related publications have been progressively acquiring more attention. Studies have been showing that low QoL is a risk factor for increased hospitalization, diminished adherence to treatment, and increased morbidity and mortality. Considering these factors, it is impossible to focus the evaluation of patients merely on the bio-physiological aspects of the diseases. Presently, QoL evaluation is an important part of the management of endocrine diseases [5-8].

References

[1] Victor C, Scambler S, Bond J, Bowling A. Being alone in later life: loneliness, social isolation and living alone. *Rev Clin Gerontol,* 2000, 10:407-17.

[2] Smith J. Well-being and health from age 70 to 100: findings from the Berlin Aging Study. *Eur Rev,* 2001, 9:461-77.

[3] Campbell A. The sense of well-being in America. New York: McGraw Hill: 1981.

[4] DeCoster, VA. Challenges of type 2 diabetes and the role of health care social workers: A neglected area of practice. *Health & Social Work,* 2001, 26:26-37.

[5] Rubin RR & Peyrot M. Quality of life and diabetes. *Diabetes/Metab Res Rev,* 1999, 15, 205-218.

[6] Fan VS et al. Using quality of life to predict hospitalization and mortality in patients with chronic obstructive pulmonary disease. *Chest, 2002*, 122:429-436.

[7] Jacobson DL. Health-related quality of life predicts survival, cytomegalovirus disease, and study retention in clinical trial participants with advanced HIV disease. *J Clin Epidemiol,* 2003, 56(9):874-8793.

[8] Westin L. Patients with ischemic heart disease: quality of life predicts long-term mortality. *Scand Cardiovasc J,* 2005, 39(1-2):50-54.

In: Quality of Life in Endocrine Diseases ISBN: 978-1-63463-911-8
Editor: Erika Cesar de Oliveira Naliato © 2015 Nova Science Publishers, Inc.

Chapter 2

Clinically Nonfunctioning Pituitary Adenomas and Quality of Life

Cristine F. Martins and Erika C. O. Naliato*
Center of Studies Ricardo A. T. Castilho of the Teresópolis Medical Association, Brazil

Abbreviations

ESS:	Epworth Sleepiness Scale
FGF:	Fibroblast growth factor
FSH:	Follicle-stimulating hormone
GH:	Growth hormone
GHRH:	Growth hormone-releasing hormone
HADS:	Hospital Anxiety and Depression Scale
HCG:	Human chorionic gonadotropin
ICP:	Intracranial pressure
LH:	Luteinizing hormone
MFI 20:	Multidimensional Fatigue Index
MR:	Magnetic resonance
NFA:	Nonfunctioning pituitary adenoma

* Correspondence to: erikanaliato@uol.com.br.

NHP:	Nottingham Health Profile
PCNA:	Proliferating cell nuclear antigen
PSQI:	Pittsburgh Sleep Quality Index
QoL-AGHDA:	Quality of Life - Assessment of Growth Hormone Deficiency in Adults
rhGH:	Recombinant human GH
SF-36:	Short Form 36
SMR:	Standardized mortality ratio

Keywords: Non-functioning pituitary adenomas, Quality of life

Clinically Nonfunctioning Pituitary Adenomas

One of the greatest difficulties in discussing nonfunctioning pituitary adenomas is that it has no universally accepted definition. Nonfunctioning adenomas were called chromophobic tumors (before the advent of immunohistochemistry), nonsecretory, or clinically silent tumors, and they name a group of tumors that do not possess a clinical syndrome resulting from hormonal hypersecretion [1]. In this work, we will adopt the term nonfunctioning pituitary adenoma (NFA).

When found in image exams performed for other reasons, the NFA is called incidentaloma. With the more frequent use of magnetic resonance (MR) due to its increasing availability in our milieu, more incidentalomas have been detected. In more recent studies, the frequency of incidentalomas among the NFA cases is around 15-25% [2, 3].

Pituitary adenomas can be classified, according to size, as microadenomas (those with a diameter inferior to 1 cm) or macroadenomas (those with a diameter equal or superior to 1 cm). Another form of classification considers the local hormonal production, where NFA are divided into secretory, when there is local production of one or more hormones, and nonsecretory, the *null-cell* [4]. The natural history of microadenomas shows us that a small nonfunctioning tumor may take around eight years to develop due to its restrictive proliferative activity [5].

The frequency of NFA varies according to the different studies, methods, and criteria [3]. Among all the pituitary adenomas, the NFA correspond to 30% [6]. It is estimated that approximately 50% of the microadenomas are nonfunctioning [7]; a frequency that increases to 80% when we analyze the macroadenomas [8, 9]. This difference may be explained by the greater facility to diagnose secretory tumors - which cause clinical symptoms in precocious phases of the tumoral development and growth in comparison to the nonsecretory, diagnosed as a result of the appearance of tumoral mass effects [3].

Hormonal Production

One of the main reasons for the absence of consensus over the definition of NFA is that, in the morphologic exam, these tumors always have cells capable of secreting pituitary hormones, which suggests the capacity of hormonal production and storage [10]. Around 86% of them present positive immunohistochemistry for at least one subunit of glycoprotein hormone, usually being positive for FSH, LH, and alpha-subunit [10]. The local production of the beta-subunits of LH, FSH, and HCG can also be found. It is considered that, with the improvement of research techniques and the growing interest for the area, more tumors will become classified as nonfunctioning [11].

Patogenesis

In effect, all pituitary tumors are originally monoclonal. Molecular studies show that the majority of the alterations common in malignant tumors are absent in the nonfunctioning ones [12]. Its pathogenesis is determined by a complex process where a genetically modified cell suffers influences of diverse factors, such as the hypothalamic hormones (growth hormone-releasing hormone - GHRH), growth factors (fibroblast growth factor - FGF), proliferating factors (proliferating cell nuclear antigen - PCNA, and KI-67), protein P53 and proto-oncogene c-erb-B2, resulting in neoplastic growth of monoclonal cells without hormonal production [11].

Prevalence

In the global population, it is estimated that the prevalence of pituitary tumors is nearly 10% [13]. These tumors reach mostly men and postmenopausal women aged between 40 and 60 years, data that probably reflect a delay in diagnosis due to the absence of pituitary hormonal hypersecretion syndromes [14]. Pituitary adenomas are rare in childhood and adolescence: less than 10% are diagnosed before the 20 years of age [5].

Clinical Manifestations

The clinical features are basically constituted of compressive effects with visual alterations, headaches, and hypopituitarism [15, 16]. The optic chiasma, due to its localization above the pituitary gland, is particularly sensitive to the compression by pituitary tumors that expand on the superior direction. The interference with the optical fibers and local vascularization causes temporal hemianopsia, which can be insidious, recurring, or remittent [17]. When the adenoma extends in the lateral direction and invades the cavernous sinus, it may affect the oculomotor nerve, causing diplopia, ptosis, and ophthalmoplegia [18]. Visual alterations are the most common symptoms of the pituitary macroadenomas, found in approximately 75% of the patients [2].

Headache is one of the most common symptoms, present in approximately 70% of the patients [2]. It occurs due to the rise of intracranial pressure (ICP) which tensions the dura mater [12]. In addition, the tumoral expansion inside the poorly flexible limits of the sella turcica stimulates the afferent fibres of the dura mater, causing pain [19].

Hypopituitarism is caused by three mechanisms: (1) compression of the pituitary stalk, (2) compression of the functioning pituitary tissue adjacent to the tumor, (3) wrapping of the hypothalamus by the adenoma. The majority of the patients with symptomatology have some degree of hypopituitarism [3].

A small or moderate elevation of serum prolactin (under 200 ng/mL) is common due to the compression of the pituitary stalk and damaging of the dopaminergic inhibition of the prolactin secretion. Despite this increase, large tumors with slight hyperprolactinemia are not prolactinomas [20], although they are responsible for symptoms similar to those caused by this kind of tumor, such as galactorrhea and hypogonadism [17].

The classic hypogonadism progresses with reduction of libido, amenorrhea, or erectile dysfunction, generating a significant impairement of the sexual life of these patients. In Brazilians, Cury et al. (2009) identified hypogonadism in 63.3% of the patients with NFA [2].

In addition to this situation, weight gain, skin dryness, astenia, intolerance to cold and exercise, reduction of cognitive capacity and depression, classic symptomatology of hypothyroidism are present in 20% of the Brazilian patients [2]. GH deficiency is present, to some extent, in nearly 85% of the patients [21].

Apoplexy is a clinical syndrome that results from the sudden hemorrhage and consequent tumoral infarction [22]. It presents itself with a sudden and excruciating headache followed by nausea and vomiting. A few hours later, a neurological deficit appears due to the compression of the optic canal or the oculomotor nerve [18]. It is rare but potentially fatal, reaching 1% of the patients with pituitary tumors. This number increases according to the size of the tumor. It is believed to happen to 10-25% of the patients with NFA [23].

Natural History

The natural course of the NFA is unknown since a great part of the nonfunctioning adenomas is treated surgically [24]. Spontaneous regression of the tumoral volume was observed in 29% of the patients and stabilization in 21% during a long term follow up study. No predicitive factors for tumoral growth were found [3]. The rare pituitary adenomas that evolve with metastasis are, in reality, originally secretory [25]. The malignization is extremely uncommon [26], despite the local invasion being a frequent phenomenon [27].

The relation with the rise in mortality due to the presence of the tumor or its treatment is unknown [28]. Despite this, there has been an increase in mortality (SMR - *standardized mortality ratio*) in patients with hypopituitarism [29,30].

Treatment

Treatment intends to improve the quality of life, alleviating the compressive symptoms, as well as preserving or improving pituitary function.

Nevertheless, the validity of different treatment modalities is still object of debate.

The most accepted therapeutic option is the endoscopic transsphenoidal surgery, recommended when tumors close to the optic chiasma are identified, with signs of hypopituitarism or with a considerable growth during clinical follow up [31]. More invasive transcranial surgery is reserved to patients with substantial suprasellar expansion or already submitted to unsuccessful endoscopic surgery, with worse prognostic [32]. Another indication for intracranial surgery is the presence of gigantic adenomas, that have no other treatment, with high mortality rates if compared to the classic macroadenomas [3].

The surgical treatment is not indicated to incidentalomas, asymptomatic NFA, small macroadenomas, or patients without clinical condition to be submitted to surgery, such as elderly people and carriers of serious underlying diseases. Expectant conduct with repetition of RM every 6 months is an option [18]. In addition to this, it remains a challenge to determine which would be the best treatment for the NFA without visual symptoms [3].

The perioperative mortality is minimal, around 1% when performed by experienced surgeons. The resolution of clinical symptoms has been documented [18]. The surgery allows the improvement of visual symptoms in 80% of patients during precocious postoperative period and immediate relief of the headache in the majority of cases [8, 33, 34, 35].

Nonetheless, the improvement of the hypopituitarism is not a consensus [18]. Some studies show a variable recovery of the pituitary function diverging from others which point out to an aggravation resulting from the surgery [35, 36, 37, 38, 39, 40, 41]. These conflicting data result from different criteria in each study, such as the definition of hypopituitarism, use of radiotherapy, and follow-up time varying from 1 week to 1 year [35]. The GH deficiency remains in 83% of patients [3].

Recurrence and complication rates vary according to the methods and must be well evaluated before the indication of treatment in order to avoid a permanent detriment of the quality of life. The long-term results of surgery vary considerably between different studies [3]. In 90% of the cases, resection of the pituitary gland is only partial [38]. There is recurrence in only 10% of patients not submitted to radiotherapy [39]. This latter therapeutic modality is infrequently used as the sole treatment of NFA for not being capable of restoring the vision and due to the ongoing improvement of the surgical techniques [40].

For the indication of radiotherapy, factors such as life expectancy, patient's wish and symptomatology must be taken into consideration. The radiotherapy treatment incurs in high rates of permanent hypopituitarism (present in 50% of the patients, in 10 years), risk of actinic lesion over the optic chiasma, and induction to other tumors [42]. Studies indicate a reduction in the post-radiotherapy life expectation; mainly due to the rise in risk of cerebrovascular diseases despite the adequate hormonal replacement [42, 43, 44]. Conversely, this therapeutic modality promotes the improvement or stabilization of the visual alterations in patients without conditions of submission to surgery with a lower recurrence rate [42].

In general, the NFA does not respond to pharmachological therapy [45]. The pharmacological treatment intends to reduce tumoral volume [24]. For that, drugs such as dopaminergic agonists and somatostatin analogues have been used. Nonetheless, they are of limited efficiency and used with restrictions [43, 44, 45, 46].

Treating pituitary dysfunction caused by the tumor itself or as a consequence of its treatment is massively important for the improvement of the quality of life. The replacement of thyroid hormones, glycocorticoids, and gonadal steroids in young adults may be necessary. Estrogenic replacement is reserved to women with exacerbation of vasomotor symptoms, such as hot flushes [47].

Hormonal replacement must be associated with evaluation of the basal levels of T4, cortisol, and testosterone in men. It must be mentioned that just one normal value of morning cortisol does not exclude the presence of deterioration of the hypothalamic-pituitary-adrenal axis [20]. Diabetes insipidus must be treated immediately after the diagnosis [47].

It has not been defined whether the administration of recombinant human GH (rhGH) for adults improves or not the prognostic of patients with hypopituitarism, which, allied to its high cost, limits its ordinary use. The improvement of quality of life with the replacement of rhGH is suggested by the increase of bone and muscular mass, reduction of fat mass, and increase of the cardiac contraction strength [42, 44, 48]. It is also known that there is an improvement of the lipidic profile of these patients after one year of therapy, independently of the level of obesity, reflecting positively in the quality of life [49].

Quality of Life

The literature is extremely scarce regarding the study of the quality of life in patients with NFA. The majority of the studies about quality of life in patients with pituitary tumors include heterogeneous groups and are not specifically focused on this type of pituitary tumor. It is a questionable strategy to compare NFA and clinically secretory tumors because they are different in many aspects [39]. NFA is more prevalent in patients older than those with secretory tumors [50]. Besides, the NFA are usually bigger and with a higher degree of hormonal deficiency [51, 52]. Despite the difference between the methods and the groups used, all the presently published studies we are aware of agree that there is reduction in the quality of life of patients with NFA [39].

In a Brazilian study done with the female population using the SF-36 questionnaire, women with NFA presented lower scores than the control ones on the subjects functional capacity, pain, general health state, vitality, and mental health. It was shown that functional capacity and vitality are related to age at the moment of the NFA diagnosis. The general and mental health were connected to the length of treatment [53].

The impact that a chronic disease, of difficult treatment and that requires the adoption of complex pharmachological management, including hormonal replacement schemes, and multiple medical consultations has a negative impact on patients' self-esteem [54].

Quality of Life Questionnaires for Patients with Nonfunctioning Pituitary Adenomas

There is no questionnaire developed exclusively for patients with NFA. The absence of a specific questionnaire is possibly owed to the small number of studies about QoL in patients with NFA. Nevertheless, the use of different questionnaires as evaluation instruments generates data, which once gathered, allow us to quantify the actual QoL of these patients [39].

The Short Form 36 (SF-36) is one of the most-used instruments in the research of QoL. It has internal consistency and external validity [55]. Its greatest limitation for the use in patients with pituitary tumors is the absence of specific questions about sexual activity, highly affected in patients with secondary hypogonadism [56]. It is composed of thirty six questions laid as a profile of eight different subgroups: functional aspect, physical capacity to perform tasks, presence and impact of the physical pain, general health, vitality, social integration, emotional aspect related to the performance of tasks, and mental health. The scores obtained are directly proportional to the QoL.

The MFI-20 questionnaire (*Multidimensional Fatigue Index*) has been developed for a complete evaluation of the fatigue experienced by the patient. There are 20 questions divided in general, physical, and mental fatigue, limitations of daily life activities, and reduction in motivation. The score obtained in the questionnaire is directly proportional to the degree of fatigue presented by the patient [39].

The HADS (*Hospital Anxiety and Depression Scale*) has 14 items with values between 1 and 4 related to aspects associated with anxiety and depression. The seriousness of the state of anxiety/depression is directly proportional to the score obtained [39].

The NHP (*Nottingham Health Profile*) is a questionnaire frequently used in patients with pituitary diseases for the evaluation of the general well-being and quality of life. It consists of thirty eight questions divided into six subgroups: pain, sleep, emotional reaction, physical mobility, and energy [39].

Hypopituitarism

The presence of multiple deficiencies of the pituitary hormones is unquestionably the predominant and independent factor for a worse QoL in patients with NFA [39, 52]. Recent findings show that this deterioration persists even long after a successful treatment [39].

Studies show a higher tendency for depression in patients with hypopituitarism when compared with patients with chronic diseases, such as Diabetes Mellitus [57]. Many of these patients present a reduction in the socioeconomic level after the diagnosis of NFA due to the interruption of their work activities [58]. There is a higher index of retirement due to disability [59], the rate of unemployment is three times higher than expected for the age, and the family income is reduced [60].

On the affective side, it has been shown that the number of married patients was 30% lower than in the general population [60]. Complaints about physical and mental fatigue are common, in addition to the reduction of libido and alterations of the sleep-wakefulness cycle. The feminine population is more affected in comparison with the control group [61].

In general, psychiatric diseases are common in patients with endocrine conditions [54]. In disagreement with this vision, Korali et al. (2003) suggest that despite the finding of a significant and constant hormonal deficiency of patients with NFA, there is no rise of risk of development of psychopathies, when these patients are compared with the population of the same gender and age. In addition, these authors did not find a relation between the incidence of mental diseases, analyzed by a scale of symptoms, and any degree of hypopituitarism or hyperprolactinemia [62].

The hypocortisolism, many times induced during the NFA treatment, may lead to astenia, cognitive deficits, anorexia, weight loss, apathy, headaches, and even coma, in rare cases [63]. These alterations generate by themselves significant loss of quality of life.

After performing interviews with NFA-diagnosed patients' relatives, Peace et al. (1997) affirmed that patients with hypopituitarism have social adjustment problems and a diminished self-evaluation capacity. These alterations occur mostly in those submitted to transsphenoidal surgery and clinical treatment when compared with those submitted to radiotherapy or transfrontal surgery [64].

In men, the testosterone deficit leads to a passive-dependent behavior with significant humor oscillations [65]. The influence of low concentrations of estrogen and progesterone in the feminine behavior is well known, causing effects similar to those of the pre-menstrual syndrome. Aggressive behavior, irritability, drop of self-esteem, and emotional lability become evident [66].

The relation between thyroid hormones and humor alterations is undeniable. Hypothyroidism leads to a depressive pattern with strong impairement of the capacity to execute tasks and the vitality [65].

Hormonal Replacement

The hormonal replacement therapy does not faithfully reproduce the hormonal profile of healthy people. And this imperfection may result in a reduced QoL even in those patients with NFA that receive hormonal replacement [67]. It is known that the GH deficiency is strongly connected to a dysfunction in learning processes, attention disturbs, and memory. Clinically, there is difficulty in evoking and retaining new information [61].

In addition, the hormonal replacement has not reached unanimity as routine treatment in patients with NFA and studies about its real impact on the QoL are not consistent [68]. There are accounts of improvement of the general well-being indexes with the use of hormonal therapy as well as placebo [69]. Conversely, double-blind studies demonstrated few or no effects on the QoL with the use of recombining GH or placebo [70, 71]. Over the last few years, the possible improvement of the patients' QoL appeared as an additional factor for the indication of the hormonal replacement therapy. Despite this, high indexes of collateral effects (varying from 24- 37%) [72, 73] limitate its everyday use [74]. The replacement therapy seems to be more efficient in patients with higher degree of hypopituitarism [75].

Sleep Disorders

Resting is one of the most important aspects for a healthy life. Biermansz et al. (2011) studied patients submitted to surgical treatment for nonfunctioning adenomas using specific questionnaires (ESS - *Epworth Sleepiness Scale*, PSQI - *Pittsburgh Sleep Quality Index*, HADS, SF-36, MFI-20), night polysomnography and 'actigraphy'. The total sleep duration (total time spent in bed during the night) was not different from the control group; nevertheless, treated patients spent more time awaken, and consequently, they possess a less efficient sleep. A difficulty of those patients in accounting for the number of hours actually slept was verified. Patients evaluated in this study related intense fatigue with physical and mental distress followed by depressive feelings and limitations of the daily activities. This is reflected on the questionnaires with high scores on MFI-20 and HADS, demonstrating the presence of classic symptoms of anxiety and depression. According to the SF-36, patients suffer with a worse physical condition that affects their social activities. In conclusion, the studied patients suffered with irregular distribution of the stages of sleep and alterations on the circadian cycle with important drop in QoL [76].

Patients previously treated by surgery also suffer from an increase in diurnal somnolence, which has no relation to age group [67]. It is believed that the rise in diurnal somnolence may be caused by the reduction of the nocturnal secretion of melatonin [77].

Clinical studies show that factors such as radiotherapy treatment and gender influence on the sleep schedule, while the duration of the sleep would be related to the presence of hypopituitarism [67].

It is believed that sleep disturbance is caused by the effects of the tumor in the supra-chiasmatic nucleus - the hypothalamic nucleus responsible for the regulation of the sleep-vigilance cycle located close to the optic chiasma [76].

Besides, the hypothalamus is also vulnerable to radiotherapy-induced lesions, which can be related to the alterations found in these patients over the post-treatment period, including in the long term [78].

Nonfunctioning Adenoma Treatment and Quality of Life

The use of post-surgery radiotherapy in the prevention of tumoral recurrence is still under debate. Dekkers et al. (2008) are defensors of the negative impact of radiation over the quality of life [3]. They believe that radiotherapy for pituitary tumors, including the nonfunctioning, is associated with a worse QoL [3, 79]. Their studies demonstrated that transsphenoidal surgery without post-surgery radiotherapy is a secure and effective strategy for NFA taking into consideration the current high indexes of cure. Even in the case of residual tumors, relapse is not observed in 87% of the patients. Some centers use radiotherapy to prevent tumoral relapse [3, 80, 81, 82, 83]. Despite this practice, relapse occurs in 2-36% of the patients who received radiation [81, 82, 84]. The possible benefit of post-surgery radiotherapy in the reduction of the indexes of long-term relapse must be balanced against the potential collateral effects, such as permanent hypopituitarism [85] and secondary cerebral tumors [86]. An expectant conduct after surgery has the advantage of postponing the possible complications of radiotherapy in patients with relapse risk. Nevertheless, in the case of relapse, radiotherapy continues to be effective to stabilize or even diminish tumoral growth [87]. With this strategy of reducing the use of radiation, the majority of the patients will not be exposed to a higher risk of complications. In addition, in those with relapse, these complications will be postponed for a few years with extension of a better quality of life [39].

The quality of life of patients submitted to radiotherapy treatment of the NFA is a controversial topic and has been amply discussed. Noad et al. (2004) analyzed the effects of radiotherapy in the cognitive function and in the QoL of patients with pituitary adenoma through the application of the SF-36 questionnaire. They concluded that the patients did not have any significant differences on the mental health and functional aspect scores after the radiotherapy treatment [88].

Page et al. (1997) studied the effects of radiotherapy on QoL in a small group of patients with NFA submitted to radiotherapy. These authors concluded that the patients treated with radiotherapy are more subjected to depression and anxiety than patients submitted to mastoid surgery [68]. Despite this, these data are not in accordance with those by Van Beek et al. (2007) who included 81 patients with NFA treated with surgery and radiotherapy followed up by a minimum period of 1 year. For the latter, the social integration, vitality, and general health (obtained by the SF-36) were significantly more compromised in the group that did not receive radiotherapy if compared with the general population. The scores related to physical activity, pain, and anxiety were not affected, being slightly better than the group that was not submitted to radiation. In their patients, the age at the surgery, the length of follow-up, the socioeconomic level, and other comorbidities were not considered relevant [67]. It is important to study other factors when analyzing the effects of radiotherapy on the QoL of patients with NFA. The indication of this modality of therapy may be considered a tendency in the analysis, since many authors indicate it for the treatment of patients with larger and more aggressive tumors. Considering this, many patients treated with radiotherapy relate high levels of vitality and less depressive symptoms besides less physical and mental fatigue. With this, it can be suggested that radiotherapy may generate an improvement in the self-evaluation of these patients [67].

On the other hand, various studies suggest that the patients with pituitary tumors continue to suffer with cognitive alterations even after a well-succeeded treatment [64, 90, 91]. McCord et al. (1997) believe that these alterations may be associated with radiotherapy [92]. Nonetheless, studies such as the one by Grattan-Smith et al. (1992) were not able to identify the specific causes for the alterations in the QoL of patients with NFA. The latter authors conducted neuropsychological tests in a group of patients with pituitary adenoma and demonstrated a drop in the capacity to execute tasks and memorization difficulties. The performance of the patients who received radiotherapy was the same as the ones treated surgically [90].

Peace et al. (1998) also showed deficits in the capacity to execute tasks in patients with pituitary tumors and attributed them to surgery and not to radiotherapy [64]. Guinan et al. (1998) found an increase of the incidence of anterograde amnesia in patients with pituitary tumors, but did not search for explanations for such evidence [91].

Conclusion

The QoL is unmistakably reduced in patients diagnosed with NFA. Many studies demonstrate that there are significant alterations in practically all types of questionnaires validated for QoL evaluation [36, 68, 76, 93].

The medical community has indicated a greater interest in the evaluation of QoL, and with this, increase the promotion of an integrated assistance with more effective treatments and a more complete follow-up. QoL became an important parameter for the therapeutic decision and, as a consequence, the number of researchers interested in the creation of new instruments of self-evaluation increased [94].

The absence of specific questionnaires for the investigation of the QoL in patients with NFA is one of the limiting factors to the furthering of their studies. With the necessity of improving these data, new questionnaires such as the QoL-AGHDA (*Quality of Life - Assessment of Growth Hormone Deficiency in Adults*) are being developed and must be tested in double-blind clinical experiments [74]. It would be important to construct a questionnaire specific for the NFA.

The WHO defines quality of life as "the individuals' perception of their position in life in the context of the cultural and values systems in which they live, and in relation to their goals, expectations, standards and concerns". This is a complex concept that values ampler parameters than the control of symptoms, reduction of mortality, and increase in life expectancy [95]. Today, it is known that it involves more than just psychological reactions, such as anxiety and depression and the neurocognitive and memory alterations. Subjective feelings, such as the perception of the physical and mental health, levels of energy and vitality are also taken into account [74]. The quality of sleep is also recognizably affected in patients with NFA [76]. Despite this, there is no specific item for the evaluation of sleep in the most-used questionnaires in almost all the studies about quality of life.

The diagnosis of pituitary adenomas without the hypersecretion syndrome is usually postponed. With this, patients suffer with symptomatology during years before receiving medical attention, which generates high expectation in relation to the treatment [16]. When present, the visual symptoms and the headache generate by themselves an important fall in the QoL of these patients. Hypopituitarism is the most serious complication and one of the most common among the pituitary tumors, being the main cause for the low QoL of these patients [39, 93].

Unfortunately, even adequate treatment is not able to provide the well-being in its entirety and normalize the life of the patients with pituitary tumors. Despite the great improvement in the visual accuracy after transsphenoidal surgery and the almost immediate relief of the headaches, it is not possible to restitute the QoL of these patients [33]. Surgical treatment revealed itself to be the most suitable for being a safe and effective procedure, reducing morbidity and avoiding the use of radiotherapy [36, 39, 92].

Radiotherapy's impact on QoL is a reason for considerable discussion between the authors. In reality, it is not possible to obtain consistent data for comparison, since there are great differences between the analyzed groups [36, 68, 93, 96]. Isolated findings suggest that patients with NFA submitted to transsphenoidal surgery associated to radiotherapy have a better perception of their condition, which promotes improvement of QoL [89].

One hypothesis to explain the restriction to the improvement in QoL of patients with NFA is the impact that a chronic disease of difficult treatment has on the self-esteem and social interaction of these patients, with frequent medical consultations, and adoption of complex pharmachological schemes [54].

References

[1] Klibanski A. Non-secretory pituitary tumors. *Endocrinol Metab Clin North Am,* 1987, 16:793-804.

[2] Cury M. L. et al. Non-functioning pituitary adenomas: clinical feature, laboratorial and imaging assessment, therapeutic management and outcome. *Arq Bras Endocrinol Metabol.*, 2009, 53:31-39

[3] Dekkers O. M., Pereira A. M., Romijn J. Treatment and Follow-Up of Clinically Nonfunctioning Pituitary Macroadenomas. *J Clin Endocrinol Metab.*, 2008, 93:3717–3726.

[4] Kovacs K., Horvath E., Ryan N., Ezrin C., et al. Null cell adenoma of the human pituitary. *Virchows Arch*, 1980, 387:165-174.

[5] Pekic S., Popovic-Brkic V. Advances is our understanding of pituitary adenoma. *European Endocrinology*, 2008, 4:57-59.

[6] Milker-Zabel S., Debus J., Thilmann C., Schlegel W., Wannenmacher, M. Fractionated stereotactically guided radiotherapy and radiosurgery in the treatment of functional and nonfunctional adenomas of the pituitary gland. *Int J Radiat Oncol Biol Phys.*, 2001, 50:1279-1286.

[7] McComb D. J., Ryan N., Horvath E., Kovacs K. Subclinical adenomas of the human pituitary. New light on old problems. *Arch Pathol Lab Med.*, 1983, 107:488 –491.

[8] Donovan L. E., Coreblum B. The natural history of the pituitary incidentaloma. *Arch Intern Med.*, 1995, 155:181–183.

[9] Sanno N., Oyama K., Tahara S., Teramoto A., Kato Y. A survey of pituitary incidentaloma in Japan. *Eur J Endocrinol.*, 2003, 149:123–127.

[10] Ferreira J. E., Mello P. A., Magalhães A. V., et al. Caracterização clínica e imunoistoquímica dos adenomas clinicamente não funcionantes de hipófise. *Arq Neuropsiquiatr.*, 2005, 63:1070-1078.

[11] Jameson J. L., Klibanski A., Black P. M., et al. Glycoprotein hormone genes are expressed in clinically nonfunctioning pituitary adenomas. *J Clin Invest.*, 1987, 80:1472-1478.

[12] Ironside J. W. Best Practice No 172: pituitary gland pathology. *J Clin Pathol.,* 2003, 56:561-568.

[13] Hall W. A., Luciano M. G., Doppman J. L., Patronas N. J., Oldfield E. H. Pituitary magnetic resonance imaging in normal human volunteers: occult adenomas in the general population. *Ann Intern Med.*, 1994, 120:817–820.

[14] Pandey P., Ojha B. K., Mahapatra A. K. Pediatric pituitary adenoma: a series of 42 patients. *J Clin Neurosci.*, 2005, 12:124-127.

[15] Comtois R., Beauregard H., Somma M., Serri O., Aris-Jilwan N., Hardy J. The clinical and endocrine outcome of transsphenoidal microsurgery of non functioning pituitary adenomas. *Cancer*, 1991, 68: 860-868.

[16] Mortini P., Losa M., Barzaghi R., Boari N., Giovanelli M., et al. Results of transsphenoidal surgery in a large series of patients pituitary adenoma. *Neurosurgery*, 2005, 56:1222-1233.

[17] Nielsen E. H., Lindholm J., Laurberg P., et al. Nonfunctioning pituitary adenoma: incidence, causes of death and quality of life in relation to pituitary function. *Pituitary*, 2007, 10:67-73.

[18] Losa M., Peretti E., Mortini P. Surgical Indications and Results for Non-functioning Pituitary Adenomas. *Eur Endocrinol.*, 2008, 4:86-89.

[19] Pascual J., Freijanes J., Berciano J., Pesquera C. Analgesic effect of octreotide in headache associated with acromegaly is not mediated by opioid mechanisms. Case report . *Pain*, 1991, 47:341-344.

[20] Thorner M. O. The anterior pituitary. In: Wilson J. *Williams textbook of endocrinology*, 9. ed. Philadelphia, USA. Saunders Elsevier; 1998:249-340.

[21] Kreutzer J., Fahlbusch R. Diagnosis and treatment of pituitary tumors. *Curr Opin Neurol.*, 2004, 17: 693-703.

[22] Cardoso E. R., Peterson E. W. Pituitary apoplexy: a review. *Neurosurgery*, 1984; 14:363-373.

[23] Nielsen, EH; Lindholm, J; Laurberg, P et al. Frequent occurrence of pituitary apoplexy in patients with nonfunctioning pituitary adenoma. *Clin Endocrinol.*, 2006, 64:319-322.

[24] Colao A., Di Somma C., Pivonello R., Faggiano A., Lombardi G., Savastano S., Lao A., et al. Medical therapy for clinically non-functioning pituitary adenomas. *Endocr Relat Cancer*, 2008, 15: 905-915.

[25] Asa S. L. The pathology of pituitary tumors. *Endocrinol Metab Clin North Am.*, 1999, 28:13-vi.

[26] Imboden P. N. E., Borruat F. X., Tribolet N., Meagher-Villemure K., Pica A., Gomez F. Nonfunctioning pituitary carcinoma. *Pituitary*, 2004, 7:149-156.

[27] Selman W. R., Laws E. R., Sheithauer B. H., Carpenter S. M. The occurrence of dural invasion in pituitary adenomas. *J Neurosurg.*, 1986, 64:402-407.

[28] Benveniste R. J., King W. A., Walsh J., Lee J. S., Delman B. N., Post K. D. Repeated transsphenoidal surgery to treat recurrent or residual pituitary adenoma. *J Neurosurg.*, 2005, 102:1004-1012.

[29] Tomlinson J. W., Holden N., Hills R. K., et al. Association between premature mortality and hypopituitarism. West Midlands Prospective Hypopituitary Study Group. *Lancet*, 2001, 357:425-431.

[30] Rosen T., Bengtsson B. A. Premature mortality due to cardiovascular disease in hypopituitarism. *Lancet*, 1990, 336:285-288.

[31] Greenman Y., Melmed S. Diagnosis and management of non functioning pituitary tumors. *Annu Rev Med.*, 1996, 47:95-106.

[32] Laws E. R., Thapar K. Pituitary surgery. *Endocrionol Metab Clin North Am.*, 1999, 28:119-131.

[33] Losa M., Mortini P., Barzaghi R., Franzin A., Giovanelli M. et al. Endocrine inactive and gonadotroph adenomas: diagnosis and management. *J Neuro-oncol.*, 2001, 54: 167–177.

[34] Dekkers O. M., de Keizer R. J., Roelfsema F., et al. Progressive improvement of impaired visual acuity during the first year after transsphenoidal surgery for non-functioning pituitary macroadenoma. *Pituitary*, 2007, 10:61–65.

[35] Losa M., Mortini P., Barzaghi R., et al. Early results of surgery in patients with non-functioning pituitary adenoma and analysis of the risk of tumour recurrence, *J Neurosurg.*, 2008, 108:525–532.

[36] Dekkers O. M., Pereira, A. M., Roelfsema F., et al. Observation alone after transsphenoidal surgery for nonfunctioning pituitary macroadenoma, *J Clin Endocrinol Metab.*, 2006, 91:1796–1801.

[37] Nomikos P., Ladar C., Fahlbusch R., Buchfelder M. Impact of primary surgery on pituitary function in patients with non-functioning pituitary adenomas- a study on 721 patients. *Acta Neurochir.*, 2004, 146:27–35.

[38] van den Bergh A. C., van den Berg G., Schoor L., et al. Immediate postoperative radiotherapy in residual nonfunctioning pituitary adenoma; beneficial effect on local control without additional negative impact on pituitary function and life expectancy. *J Rad Oncol Biol Phys.*, 2007, 68:986-991.

[39] Dekkers O. M., van der Klaauw A. A., Pereira A. M., et al. Quality of life is decreased after treatment for nonfunctioning pituitary macroadenoma. *J Clin Endocrinol Metab.*, 2006, 91:3364–3369.

[40] Brada M., Jankowska P. Radiotherapy for pituitary adenoma. *Endocrinol Metab Clin N Am.*, 2008, 37:263-275.

[41] Alameda C., Lucas T., Pineda E., et al., Experience in management of 51 non-functioning pituitary adenomas: indications for post-operative radiotherapy. *J Endocrinol Invest.*, 2005, 28:18–22.

[42] Cunha Neto M., Musolino M., Bronstein M. D. Manuseio dos adenomas hipofisários clinicamente não-funcionantes. In: Vilar L. *Endocrinologia Clínica.* 2ª ed. Rio de Janeiro, Brazil: MEDSI; 2000: 68-79.

[43] Molich M. E. Nonfunctioning pituitary tumors and incidentalomas. *Endocrionol Metab Clin North Am.*, 2008, 37:151-171.

[44] Chanson P. Traitement des adénomes hypophysaires. *Presse Med.*, 1998, 27:2077-2097.

[45] Sassolas G., Trouillas J., Treluyer C., Perrin G. Management of nonfunctioning pituitary adenomas. *Acta Endocrinol (Copenh)*, 1993; 129:121-126.

[46] Bevan J. S., Webster J., Burke C. W., Scanlon M. F., et al. Dopamine agonists and pituitary tumor shinkrage. *Endocrine Rev.*, 1992, 13:220-240.

[47] Naves L. Adenomas Hipofisários Clinicamente Não-Funcionantes. In: Villar L (eds). *Endocrinologia Clínica*, 4. Ed.. Rio de Janeiro, Brasil:Guanabara Koogan; 2009:101-112.

[48] Chanson P., Salenave S. Diagnosis and treatment of pituitary adenomas. *Minerva Endocrinol.*, 2004, 29:239-273.

[49] Abrams P., Boquete H., Fideleff H., et al. GH replacement in hypopituitarism improves lipid profile and quality of life independently of changes in obesity variables. *Eur J Endocrinol.*, 2008, 159:825–832.

[50] Mindermann T., Wilson C. B. Age-related and gender-related occurrence of pituitary adenomas. *Clin Endocrinol.*, 1994, 41:359-364.

[51] Biermasz N. R., van Thiel S. W., Pereira A. M., et al. Decreased quality of life in patients with acromegaly despite long-term cure of growth hormone excess. *J Clin Endocrinol Metab.*, 2004, 89: 5369-5376.

[52] van Aken M. O., Pereira A. M., Biermasz N. R., et al. Quality of life in patients after long-term biochemical cure of Cushing's disease. *J Clin Endocrinol Metab.*, 2005, 90:3279-3286.

[53] Ballarini M., Naliato E. C. O., Loureiro C. R., et al. Estudo da qualidade de vida em mulheres com macroadenomas hipofisários não-funcionantes e macroprolactinomas. *Arq Bras Endocrinol Metabol.*, 2008, 52:P11.

[54] Perreira Neto A. Pressão intra-selar media, cefaléia, qualidade de vida e prolactina sérica. Estudo prospectivo realizado em 25 pacientes operados consecutivamente no Hospital Universitário de Brasília (DF). 164p, 2006.

[55] Tepper S. A six-term short-form survey for mensuring headache impact: the HIT-6. *Qual Life Res.*, 2003, 12:963-974.

[56] Johnson M. D., Woodburn C. J., Vance M. L. Quality of life in patients with pituitary adenoma. *Pituitary*, 2003, 6:81-87.

[57] Lynch S., Merson S., Beshyah S. A., et al. Psychiatric morbidity in adults with hypopituitarism. *J R Soc Med.*, 1994, 87:445-447.

[58] Rikken B., Van Bussbacht J., Le Cressie S., et al. Imparied social status of growth hormone deficient adults as compared to controls with short or normal stature. *Clin Endocrinol.*, 1995, 43: 205-211.

[59] Rosén T., Wilrén L., Wilhelsen L., Wiklund I., Bengtsson B. A. Decreased psychological well-being in adult patients with growth hormone deficiency. *Clin Endocrinol.*, 1994, 40:111-116.

[60] Dean H. J., McTaggart T. L., Fish D. G., Friesen H. G. The educational, vocational and marital status of GH deficient adults treated with growth hormone in childhood. *Am Dis Child.*, 1985, 139:1100-1110.

[61] Baird A., Sullivan T., Zafar S., Rock J. Quality of life in patients with pituitary tumors. A preliminary study. *Qual Manag Heath Care*, 2003;12:97-105.

[62] Korali Z., Wittchen H. U., Pfister H., Hofler M., Oefelein W., Stalla G. K. Are patients with pituitary adenomas at an increased risk of mental disorders? *Acta Psychiatr Scand.*, 2003, 107:60–68.

[63] Heald A. H., Ghosh S., Bray S., et al. Long-term negative impact on quality of life in patients with successfully treated Cushing's disease. *Clin Endocrinol.*, 2004, 61:458-65.

[64] Peace K. A., Orme S. M., Sebastian J. P., et al. Cognitive dysfunction in patients with pituitary tumor who have been treated with transfrontal or transsphenoidal surgery or medication. *Clin Endocrinol.*, 1998, 49:391-396.

[65] Burman P., Deijen J. B. Quality of life and cognitive function in patients with pituitary insufficiency. *Psychoter Psychosom.*, 1998, 67:154-157.

[66] Fink G., Sumner B. E., Rosie R., Grace O., Quinn J. P. Estrogen control of central monoamission: Effect on mood, mental state and memory. *Cell Mol Neurobiol.*, 1996, 16:325-344.

[67] van der Klaauw A. A., Dekkers O. M., Pereira A. M., van Kralingen K. W., Romijn J. A. Increased daytime somnolence despite normal sleep patterns in patients treated fornonfunctioning pituitary macroadenoma. *J Clin Endocrinol Metab.*, 2007, 92:3898-3903.

[68] Page R. C., Hammersley M. S., Burke C. W., Wass J. A. An account of the quality of life of patients after treatment for non-functioning pituitary tumors. *Clin Endocrinol.*, 1997, 46:401–406.

[69] Holmes S. J., Shalet S. M. Factors influencing the desire for long-term growth hormone replacement in adults. *Clin Endocrinol.*, 1995, 43:151-157.

[70] Beshyah S. A., Henderson A., Niththyananthan R., et al. The effects of short and long-term growth hormone replacement therapy in hypopituitary adults on lipid metabolism and carbohydrate tolerance. *J Clin Endocrinol Metab.*, 1995, 80:356-363.

[71] Wallymahmed M. E., Foy P., Shaw D., Hutcheon R., Edwards R. H., MacFarlane I. A., et al. Quality of life, body composition and muscle strength in adult growth hormone deficiency: the influence of growth hormone replacement therapy for up to 3 years. *Clin Endocrinol.*, 1997, 47:439–446.

[72] Bengtsson B. A., Eden S., Lonn L., et al.Treatment of adults with growth hormone (GH) deficiency with recombinant human GH. *J Clin Endocrinol Metab.*, 1993, 76:309 –317.

[73] Attanasio A. F., Lamberts S. W., Matranga A. M., et al. Adult growth hormone (GH)-deficient patients demonstrate heterogeneity between

childhood onset and adult onset before and during human GH treatment. Adult Growth Hormone Deficiency Study Group. *J Clin Endocrinol Metab.*, 1997, 82:82–88.

[74] Barkan A. L. The "Quality of Life-Assessment of Growth Hormone Deficiency in Adults" Questionnaire: Can It Be Used to Assess Quality of Life in Hypopituitarism? *J Clin Endocrinol Metab.*, 2001, 86:1905-1907.

[75] Burman P., Broman J. E., Hetta J., et al. Quality of life in adults with growth hormone (GH) deficiency: response to treatment with recombinant human GH in a placebo controlled 21 month trial. *J Clin Endocrinol Metab.*, 1995, 80:3585-3590.

[76] Biermasz N. R., Joustra S. D., Donga E., et al. Patients previously treated for nonfunctioning pituitary macroadenomas have disturbed sleep characteristics, circadian movement rhythm, and subjective sleep quality. *J Clin Endocrinol Metab.*, 2011, 96:1524-32.

[77] Müller H. L., Handwerker G., Gebhardt U., Muller H. L., et al. Melatonin treatment in obese patients with childhood craniopharyngioma and increased daytime sleepiness. *Cancer Causes Control*, 2006, 17:583–589.

[78] Toogood A. A. Endocrine consequences of brain irradiation. *Growth Horm IGF Res.*, 2003, 14(Suppl A):S118–S124.

[79] Erfurth E. M., Bülow B., Svahn-Tapper G., et al. Risk factors for cerebrovascular deaths in patients operated and irradiated for pituitary tumors. *J Clin Endocrinol Metab.*, 2002, 87:4892–4899.

[80] Arafah B. M., Nekl K. E., Gold R. S., Selman W. R., et al. Dynamics of prolactin secretion in patients with hypopituitarism and pituitary macroadenomas. *J Clin Endocrinol Metab.*, 1995, 80: 3507–3512.

[81] Karavitaki N., Thanabalasingham G., Shore H. C., et al. Do the limits of serum prolactin in disconnection hyperprolactinaemia need re-definition? A study of 226 patients with histologically verified non-functioning pituitary macroadenoma. *Clin Endocrinol.,* 2006, 65:524–529.

[82] Kerrison J. B. Stages of improvement in visual fields after pituitary tumor resection. *Am J Ophthalmol.*, 2000, 130:813–820.

[83] Jakobsson K. E. Dynamics of visual improvement following chiasmal decompression. Quantitative pre- and postoperative observations. *Acta Ophthalmol Scand.*, 2002, 80:512–516.

[84] Dekkers O. M., Hammer S., de Keizer R. J. et al. The natural course of non-functioning pituitary macro-adenomas. *Eur J Endocrinol.*, 2007, 156:217–224.

[85] Cohen A. R., Cooper P. R., Kupersmith M. J., Flamm E. S., Ransohoff J. Visual recovery after transsphenoidal removal of pituitary adenomas. *Neurosurgery*, 1985, 17:446–452.

[86] Freda P. U., Wardlaw S. L. Clinical review 110: diagnosis and treatment of pituitary tumors. *J Clin Endocrinol Metab.*, 1999, 84:3859–3866.

[87] Yamada S., Ohyama K., Taguchi M., et al. A study of the correlation between morphological findings and biological activities in clinically nonfunctioning pituitary adenomas. *Neurosurgery*, 2007, 61:580–584.

[88] Noad R., Narayanan K. R., Howlett T., Lincoln N. B., Page R. C. Evaluation of the effect of radiotherapy for pituitary tumors on cognitive function and quality of life. *Clin Oncol.*, 2004, 16:233-237.

[89] van Beek A. P., van den Bergh A. C., van den Berg L. M., et al. Radiotherapy is not associated with reduced quality of life and cognitive function in patients treated for nonfunctioning pituitary adenoma. *Int J Radiat Oncol Biol Phys.*, 2007, 68:986-991.

[90] Grattan-Smith P. J., Morris L., Shores E. A. Batchelor J., Sparks R. S. Neuropsychological abnormalities in patients with pituitary tumors. *Acta Neurol Scand.*, 1992, 86:626-631.

[91] Guinan E. M., Lowy C., Stanhope N., Lewis P. D., Kopelman M. D. Cognitive effects of pituitary tumors and their treatments: Two case studies and an investigation of 90 patients. *J Neurol Neurosurg Psychiatry*, 1998, 65:870-876.

[92] McCord M. W., Buatti J. M., Fennell E. M., et al. Radiotherapy for pituitary adenoma: Long-term outcome and sequelae. *Int J Radiat Oncol Biol Phys.*, 1997, 39:437-444.

[93] Santos A., Resminia E., Martineza M. A., et al. Quality of life in patients with pituitary tumors. *Curr Opin Endocrinol Diabetes Obes.*, 2009, 16:299-303.

[94] Pennacchini M. A brief history of the Quality of Life: its use in medicine and in philosophy. *Clin Ter.*, 2011, 162:99-103.

[95] Yeng L.T., Teixeira M. J., Romano M. A., Greve J. M. D., Kaziyama H. H. S. Avaliação funcional da dor do doente com dor crônica. *Rev Med.*, 2001, 1:443-473.

[96] Caron P. Clinically non functioning pituitary adenomas and gonadotroph-cell adenomas. *Presse Med.*, 2009, 38:103-106.

In: Quality of Life in Endocrine Diseases ISBN: 978-1-63463-911-8
Editor: Erika Cesar de Oliveira Naliato © 2015 Nova Science Publishers, Inc.

Chapter 3

Prolactinoma and Quality of Life

Erika C. O. Naliato [*] ***and Elza F. S. Cerqueira***
Center of Studies Ricardo A. T. Castilho of the Teresópolis Medical Association, Brazil

Abbreviations

CT: computed tomography
DA: dopaminergic agonists
FSH: follicle-stimulating hormone
GnRH: gonadotropin-releasing hormone
LH: luteinizing hormone
MR: magnetic resonance
QoL: quality of life

Introduction

Pituitary tumors represent 10 to 15% of the intracranial tumors, and their prevalence in autopsy studies is around 27%. Prolactinoma, pituitary tumor producer of prolactin, is the most common, between 40% to 60% of all

[*] Correspondence to: erikanaliato@uol.com.br

adenomas in this region, and it is estimated the occurrence of 500 new cases/1.000.000 inhabitants/year [1].

Prolactinoma, lactotrophic adenoma or prolactin secretory cells adenoma, is considered the most frequent type of hyperfunctional pituitary adenoma, corresponding to almost 30% of the cases. The lesions range from small microadenomas to large expansible tumors alongside significant mass effects [1].

The main functions of prolactin are the induction of lactation and inhibition of the reproductive function. In addition, studies demonstrate that this hormone produced by the anterior pituitary is also capable of influencing metabolism, osmoregulation, fetal and perinatal growth, and even carcinogenesis [2].

Pituitary microadenomas are classified as prolactinomas when they develop with prolactin levels above 60 ng/mL and hypogonadotrophic hypogonadism associated to a pituitary image compatible with an adenoma. In macroadenomas, prolactin levels are above 100 ng/mL [1]. Regarding size, we classify the tumor according to computed tomography (CT) image or magnetic resonance (MR): microadenomas - size inferior to 1 cm; or macroadenomas - size equal or superior to 1 cm [3].

Approximately 90% of the prolactinomas are small and intrasellar, more frequent in women of fertile age, and among the most common consequences is hypogonadism, which leads to infertility [4]. The impossibility of reproduction is anguishing for the couples, especially for the women who wish to get pregnant. Sometimes questionable information, originating from varied sources, say that women with prolactinoma should not get pregnant or breast feed, which may lead the patient to frustrating moments in her personal life, which directly affects her well-being and quality of life (QoL) [5].

Prolactinoma

The prolactin, as other polypeptide hormones, has pulsatile secretion which in young individuals of both genders is characterized by short episodic patterns at awakening that increase during the night [6].

The hyperprolactinemia interferes with the hypothalamic-pituitary-ovary axis in various levels and is responsible for near 1/3 of all the cases of female infertility due to the interruption of the secretion of the hypothalamic gonadotropin-releasing hormone (GnRH), inhibiting the liberation of luteinizing (LH) and follicle-stimulating (FSH) hormones, and consequently altering the gonadal steroidogenesis [4].

The real prevalence of hyperprolactinemia is difficult to be established, however, it is estimated that, among women with reproductive disorders, near 15% have anovulation, while 43% of the ones that have anovulation and galactorrhea have hyperprolactinemia [7, 8]. Since hyperprolactinemia is usually associated with anovulation and the prolactinomas have a higher incidence in the 3rd and 4th decades of life, these tumors are an important cause of infertility.

The diagnosis of the prolactinoma is based on the presence of galactorrhea and symptoms and signs deriving of hypogonadism (menstrual irregularity, infertility, erectile dysfunction) associated to maintained hyperprolactinemia and a tumoral image (adenoma) in the pituitary computed tomography (CT) or magnetic resonance (MR). The majority of prolactinomas in women are microprolactinomas (95%), while the prevalence of macroprolactinomas is higher in men [9].

The treatment of hyperprolactinemia restores the ovulation in 80 to 90% of the cases [10]. Pituitary microsurgery and the availability of use of dopaminergic agonists (DA) bromocriptine and cabergoline (derivatives of the ergot that bind to the D2 dopamine receptors and stimulate them in both the normal and tumoral lactotrophes) resulted in a great progress in the treatment of prolactinomas and made clinical treatment the gold standard in the majority of cases, independent of the size and degree of invasion [11].

DA treatment normalizes the levels of prolactinoma in 75 to 85% of patients, restores the ovulation in 80 to 90% of women with micro or macroprolactinomas, and reduces tumoral growth in 25 to 68% of the cases [10].

The DA most frequently used in our country is bromocriptine which is in the market for a longer time and is administered orally, daily, in doses that vary from 1.25 to 10 mg/day.

Bromocriptine may present collateral effects, mostly on the gastrointestinal tract, that lead to persistent intolerance, many times mistaken for resistance, observed in near 10% of the patients. Since this agonist is the older in terms of market availability, it is the one with the greatest number of publications ensuring effectiveness and absence of fetal physical malformations, when its use is necessary during pregnancy [11, 12].

Cabergoline has a more prolonged action due to its long half-life, being administered orally in doses of 0.125 to 4.0 mg/week. This agent has a much lower incidence of collateral effects, and the patients fit themselves to the therapeutic schemes more easily [11]. When used in the treatment of prolactinomas, it presents better results than bromocriptine and is the drug considered the top-of the-line for the use in prolactinomas by the recommendations of the consensus published in February 2011 by the American and European Endocrinology Societies [12].

Higher incidence of fetal deformations, ectopic gestation, prematurity, or abortions than in general population were not described [1, 4, 8, 11]. Nonetheless, the guidance of the American and European Organizations (*The Endocrine Society, The European Society of Endocrinology* e *The Pituitary Society*) still advises the use of bromocriptine as the DA of choice for women who intend to get pregnant [12, 13].

Other DA such as pergolide and quinagolide are not normally used in our area. Surgery is reserved to cases of resistance to DA, failure to commit to clinical treatment, and less frequently, complications such as liquorice fistula. Radiotherapy does not show good results; it is indicated in the few cases of clinical treatment failure due to resistance and, especially, invasive tumors [14].

With treatment, the reduction in the size of the tumor is usually fast. In some patients, it occurs in 1 or 2 weeks, but the greater reduction happens during the first three months of treatment. Nevertheless, in a minority (25%), the tumor reduction is slower, taking from 6 months to up to 1 year [12]. In macroprolactinomas, visual deficit and vision improvement occur in 90% of the affected patients during the first 24 to 72 hours, and the vision continues to improve for several months [14].

Prolactin does not exercise a fundamental role for the maintenance of the life of the individual. Conversely, the consequences of a persistent elevation of the levels of this hormone are easily noticeable, both in women and men. Besides the most evident effects over the reproductive function (amenorrhea, infertility) and bone metabolism [15, 16], alterations of the PRL secretion have been related to disturbance of appetite [17], insulin resistance [18], obesity [19, 20], and glucose intolerance [19, 21]. These alterations induced by the hyperprolactinemia, allied to the effects of the tumoral mass, may cause the impairment of QoL in patients with prolactinoma.

Quality of Life

Although the literature contains various works about QoL in hypothalamic and pituitary tumors [22, 23, 24], specific data about patients with prolactinoma are still very scarce.

In contrast to what is observed in other endocrinopathies, such as acromegaly, growth hormone deficiency, and hypogonadism, there are no QoL questionnaires specifically elaborated for patients with prolactinoma or hyperprolactinemia. Due to this lack of specific questionnaires, the evaluation of patients with prolactinoma is accomplished with unspecific instruments, such as the *Short-Form Health Survey* (SF-36) [25, 26].

The diagnosis of a tumor located in the cranial region may cause a devastating emotional impact [27]. Johnson et al. (2003) studied patients with pituitary tumors (prolactinomas, acromegaly, Cushing disease, and nonfunctioning tumors) using the SF-36 questionnaire [25]. They verified that in the four types of pituitary adenomas, patients presented reduction of QoL. The study revealed specific data of patients recently diagnosed with prolactinoma who presented reduction of QoL mostly in the mental scales (social and emotional aspects and mental health). Being a sectional type of study, it was not possible to evaluate the influence of the hyperprolactinemia control and the reduction of the tumoral volume on the QoL of these patients.

The hyperprolactinemia may increase the hypothalamic tonus generating a positive retro-feeding system where prolactin increases the secretion of opioids, which by consequence increases the secretion of prolactin itself [27]. This hormone may act on the central nervous system causing behavioral alterations, such as the inhibition of sexual behavior, the disturbance of pain sensibility, the increase of learning capacity, and the reduction of the latency period for the maternal behavior [27]. It has been suggested that patients with hyperprolactinemia have a higher prevalence of depression and headache, even in the absence of demonstrable pituitary tumors [27].

Naliato et al. (2008) evaluated the QoL of women with microprolactinoma treated with DA through the SF-36 questionnaire, dividing them into two groups according to the control of the hyperprolactinemia (normal *versus* elevated prolactin) and comparing the patients with a control group. The patients presented lower scores than the control group in the eight categories of the SF-36 (functional capacity, physical aspect, pain, general health state, vitality, social and emotional aspects, and mental health). When the patients with normal and elevated prolactin levels were compared, the second group presented lower scores in all categories, except the physical aspect. The patients' scores were inversely associated with the prolactin levels. The authors drew attention to the importance of the establishment of a good control over the prolactin levels in order to avoid the reduction the QoL in patients with prolactinoma. Nonetheless, the QoL of those with normal prolactin levels was significantly inferior to the control group, which suggests that additional factors may influence the QoL of patients with prolactinoma [26]. The presence of previous psychological disturbs might justify these results [27].

Peace et al. (1997) evaluated the influence of modalities of treatment in the QoL of individuals with pituitary adenomas. The authors concluded that patients treated pharmacologically or through transsphenoidal surgery suffered from humor disturbance and social maladjustment [22]. As cited before, these modalities of treatment are the most used for prolactinomas.

The length of the pituitary tumoral disease was considered a relevant influence by Peace et al. (1997) [22]. This data was not confirmed by the study of Naliato et al. (2008) [26].

Final Considerations

Specific data about QoL in patients with prolactinoma is still very scarce. Additionally, there are no QoL questionnaires specifically elaborated for patients with prolactinoma or hyperprolactinemia.

Studies have shown a reduction of QoL in patients with prolactinoma, mostly in the mental scales (social and emotional aspects and mental health). Patients with hyperprolactinemia have a higher prevalence of depression and headache, even in the absence of demonstrable pituitary tumors. QoL may be affected by PRL levels, since it has been noticed that patients with prolactinoma that remain with elevated levels of PRL present lower QoL than the ones in whom adequate biochemical control is established.

References

[1] Vaisman M., Conceição F. L., Vieira Neto L. et al. *Prolactinomas: Rotinas diagnósticas e terapêuticas:* Serviço de Endocrinologia do Hospital Universitário Clementino Fraga Filho. São Paulo: Editora Altheneu, 2009, 15-25.

[2] Freemark M., Driscoll P., Maaskant R., Petryk A., Kelly P. A. Ontogenesis of prolactin receptors in the human fetus in early gestation - Implications for tissue differentiation and development. *J Clin Invest.*, 1997, 99:1107-1117.

[3] Horseman N. D. Prolactin. In DeGroot LJ; Jameson JL (ed). *Endocrinology*. 4th ed. Philadelphia, Pennsylvania, USA: W.B. Saunders Company; 2001:209-220.

[4] Schlechte J. A. Prolactinomas. *N Engl J Med.*, 2003, 349: 2035-41.

[5] Fleenor D., Oden J., Kelly P. A. et al. Roles of the lactogens and somatogens in perinatal and postnatal metabolism and growth: Studies of a novel mouse model combining lactogen resistance and growth hormone deficiency. *Endocrinology,* 2005, 146:103-112.

[6] Schweizer F. W., Kim M. H., Malarkey W. B. The diurnal variations of serum prolactin levels before and during pregnancy in normal and hyperprolactinemic patients. *Am J Obstet Gynecol.*, 1984, 149(4): 367-71.

[7] Imran S. A., Ur E., Clarke D. B. Managing prolactin-secreting adenomas during pregnancy. *Can Fam Physician,* 2007, 53(4):653-658.

[8] Molich M. E. Pituitary tumors and pregnancy. *Growth Horm IGF Res.,* 2003, 13:S38-S44.

[9] Braucks G. R., Naliato E. C. O., Tabet A. L. O., Gadelha M. R., Violante A. H. D. Aspectos Clínicos e Terapêuticos de Prolactinomas em Homens. *Arq Neuropsiquiatr.*, 2003, 61(4): 1004-1010.

[10] Kharlip J., Salvatori R., Yenokyan G., Wand G. S. Recurrence of Hyperprolactinemia after Withdrawal of Long-Term Cabergoline Therapy. *J Clin Endocrinol Metab.*, 2009, 94: 2428–2436.

[11] Bronstein M. D. Prolactinomas and Pregnancy. *Pituitary,* 2005, 8:31-38.

[12] Melmed S., Casanueva F. F., Hoffman A. R. et al. Diagnosis & Treatment of Hyperprolactinemia: An Endocrine Society Clinical Practice Guideline. *J Clin Endocrinol Metab.*, 2011, 96:273–288.

[13] Bronstein M. D., Paraiba D. B., Jallad R. S. Management of Pituitary Tumors in Pregnancy – *Nature Rev/Endocrinology*, 2011, 7:301-310.

[14] Randeva H. S., Davis M., Prelevic G. M. Prolactinoma and pregnancy. *Br J Ob Gynecol.*, 2000, 107:1064-1068.

[15] Colao A., Di Somma C., Loche S. et al. Prolactinomas in adolescents: persistent bone loss after 2 years of prolactin normalization. *Clin Endocrinol.*, 2000, 52:319-327.

[16] Naliato E. C. O., Farias M. L. F., Braucks G. R., Costa F. S. R., Zylberberg D., Violante A. H. D. Prevalence of osteopenia in men with prolactinoma. *J Endocrinol Invest.*, 2005, 28:12-17.

[17] Carruba M. O., Ricciardi S., Müller E. E., Mantegazza P. Anoretic effect of lisuride and other ergot derivatives in the rat. *Eur J Pharmacol.,* 1980, 64:133-141.

[18] Landgraf R., Leurs-Landgraf M. M. C., Weissmann A, Hörl R., Von Werder K., Scriba P. C. Prolactin: A diabetogenic hormone. *Diabetologia.*, 1977, 13:99-104.

[19] Cincotta A. H., Schiller B. C., Meier A. H. Bromocriptine inhibits the seasonally occurring obesity, hyperinsulinemia, insulin resistance, and impaired glucose tolerance in the Syrian hamster, *Mesocricetus auratus. Metabolism*, 1991, 40:639-644.

[20] Greenman Y., Tordjman K., Stern N. Increased body weight associated with prolactin secreting pituitary adenomas: Weight loss with normalization of prolactin levels. *Clin Endocrinol.*, 1998, 48:547-553.

[21] Barnett A. H., Chapman C., Gailer K., Hayter C. J. Effect of bromocriptine on maturity onset diabetes. *Postgrad Med J.*, 1980, 56:11-14.

[22] Peace K. A., Orme S. M., Sebastian J. P., Thompson A. R., Barnes S., Ellis A., Belchetz P. E. The effect of treatment variables on mood and social adjustment in adult patients with pituitary disease. *Clin Endocrinol (Oxf).*, 1997, 46(4):445-50.

[23] Van Aken M. O., Pereira A. M., Biermasz N. R., van Thiel S. W., Hoftijzer H. C., Smit J. W., Roelfsema F., Lamberts S. W., Romijn J. A. Quality of life in patients after long-term biochemical cure of Cushing's disease. *J Clin Endocrinol Metab.*, 2005, 90(6):3279-86.

[24] Dekkers O. M., van der Klaauw A. A., Pereira A. M., Biermasz N. R., Honkoop P. J., Roelfsema F., Smit J. W., Romijn J. A. Quality of life is decreased after treatment for nonfunctioning pituitary macroadenoma. *J Clin Endocrinol Metab.*, 2006, 91(9):3364-9.

[25] Johnson M. D., Woodburn C. J., Vance M.L. Quality of life in patients with a pituitary adenoma. *Pituitary*, 2003, 6(2):81-7.

[26] Naliato E. C. O., Violante A. H. D., Caldas D. et al. Quality of life in women with microprolactinoma treated with dopamine agonists. *Pituitary*, 2008, 11:247-254.

[27] Sobrinho L. G., Nunes M. C. P., Calhaz-Jorge C., Afonso A. M., Pereira M. C., Santos M. A. Hyperprolactinemia in women with paternal deprivation during childhood. *Obstet Gynecol.*, 1984, 64:465-468.

In: Quality of Life in Endocrine Diseases ISBN: 978-1-63463-911-8
Editor: Erika Cesar de Oliveira Naliato © 2015 Nova Science Publishers, Inc.

Chapter 4

Quality of Life in Acromegaly and Growth Hormone Deficiency

Jordan C. Moura and Erika C. O. Naliato*
Center of Studies Ricardo A. T. Castilho of the Teresópolis Medical Association, Brazil

Abbreviations

AcroQol:	Acromegaly Quality of Life Questionnaire
ACTH:	Adrenocorticotropic Hormone
BMI:	Body Mass Index
CET:	Cranial-Encephalic Traumatism
EQ 5-D:	EuroQoL
GH:	Growth Hormone
GHD:	Growth Hormone Deficiency
GHRH:	Growth Hormone Releasing Hormone
GHRP:	Growth Hormone-Releasing Peptide
IGF-1:	Insulin-Like Growth Factor - 1
NHP:	Nottingham Health Profile
OGTT:	Oral Glucose Tolerance Test
PGWBS:	Psychological General Wellbeing Schedule
QoL:	Quality of Life

* Correspondence to: erikanaliato@uol.com.br.

QoL-AGHDA:	QOL-Assessment of Growth Hormone Deficiency in Adults
QLS^{M}-H:	Questions on Life Satisfaction Modules
SF-36:	Short-Form Health Survey
SSS:	Signs and Symptoms Scores
TSH:	Thyroid Stimulating Hormone

Introduction

Growth hormone (GH) acts by mediating the growth of diverse tissues and promoting several metabolic functions through the whole body [1]. Hypothalamic stimulation mediated by GHRH (*GH releasing hormone*) is necessary for the release of this hormone [2, 3]. GHRH stimulates the anterior pituitary to liberate GH in the blood stream [2, 3].

The sexual steroids are one of the many stimulating factors to the liberation of the GHRH; considering this, we can understand the fast growth that occurs during puberty. There are other stimulating factors, such as deep sleep, alpha-adrenergic action, acetylcholine action, stress, and hypoglycemia [4, 5]. As a counterpart to the stimulating factors, there are the inhibiting factors to the secretion of GH, such as obesity, beta-adrenergic action, hyperglycemia, hypothyroidism, and IGF-1 (insulin-like growth factor) [6, 7].

IGF-1 is liberated by diverse tissues through the stimulus of GH itself, where the hepatic production is its main source. IGF-1 acts in a synergic way with GH; and in reality, it is the hormone that will link itself to the receptors located on the target-tissues, inducing cell and tissue growth. Despite that, IGF-1 inhibits the release of GH by promoting a negative *feed-back*, inhibiting the hypothalamic release of GHRH [1].

When there is no organic or exogenous alteration modifying the GNRH-GH-IGF-1 axis, the individual grows and develops in a satisfactory manner. However, there are two forms of destabilization of this axis. On one side, GH secretion increases and, on the other, the reduction of the liberation of this hormone occurs, named respectively, acromegaly and GH deficiency [1].

Acromegaly

Acromegaly is produced in more than 95% of cases by GH-secreting pituitary adenomas; the other 5% or less are a result of ectopic pituitary adenomas, such as in pituitary remnants on the sphenoid sinus, petrous temporal bone, in the nasopharynx cavity, or in the suprasellar region as well as by GH secretion from the intra-mesentery pancreas islets, and by a non-Hodgkin lymphoma [1, 8, 9]. These 5% also include cases of acromegaly due to GHRH secretion by bronchial carcinomas, pancreatic cells carcinomas, pancreatic and gastrointestinal carcinoids, small cells pulmonary carcinomas, adrenal adenomas, pheochromocytomas, medulla pituitary carcinomas, endometrium and breast cancer [1, 8, 9]. Acromegaly equally affects men and women and may happen at any age, its appearance being more common on the fourth and fifth generations of life [1]. The prevalence of this disease is 38 to 69/1,000,000 individuals, and its incidence is around 5/1,000,000 [1].

The diagnosis of acromegaly is based on the rise of GH and IGF-1 levels associated with a clinical state resulting from the increase of action of these hormones on the diverse tissues of the body, possibly causing the alterations described in Table 1. One incidental evaluation of GH level lower than 0.4 ng/mL dismisses the diagnosis of acromegaly [10]. Around 90% of the patients present GH levels higher than 10 ng/mL [1]. Random samples have little value for the diagnosis of acromegaly since GH secretion is pulsatile, varying between 5 to 500 ng/mL, with a mean of 50 ng/mL [1]. In serialized samples, 50 to 70% of patients may present undetectable GH values, and normal individuals may reach peaks of up to 30 ng/mL [1, 11]. With this, patients with acromegaly may have variations of GH levels in certain moments during the day within the limits of normality.

As IGF-1 is stimulated by GH and does not have circulating values as variable as the latter, the evaluation of IGF-1 levels may be a good screening exam for acromegaly since the elevated GH levels cause elevated IGF-1 levels [1]. Despite that, there are more specific exams for the diagnosis of this disease.

The gold standard for the diagnosis of acromegaly is the measurement of GH level after the oral glucose tolerance test (OGTT), in which GH must be measured every 30 minutes during 2 hours after the ingestion of 75 g of anhydrous glucose [10]. In individuals without acromegaly, a reduction of the GH values to less than 1 ng/mL is observed [10]. Despite that, in acromegaly the GH values may have a subtle fall or even a paradoxical rise [9].

Table 1. Effects of the long term exposition to GH and IGF-1

Bones and joints	Peripheral alterations, gigantism, prognathism, arthritis, osteopenia, vertebral fractures, carpal tunnel syndrome
Heart	Cardiomyopathy, hypertension, arrhythmia
Skin	Rise of skin oiliness, verruca
Pancreas	Resistance to insulin, diabetes
Lung	Sleep apnea
Kidney	Hydric retention, aldosterone rise, kidney failure
Thyroid	Goiter
Gonads	Hypogonadism
Muscle	Proximal myopathy
Colon	Polyposis
Fat	Lipolysis
Visceromegaly	Tongue, thyroid, salivary glands, liver, spleen, kidney, prostate

Adapted from MELMED & KLEINBERG, 2008.

Since 95% of the acromegaly cases are a result of pituitary adenomas, after the biochemical diagnosis, the execution of a pituitary magnetic resonance with contrast is necessary for the detection of the adenoma, evaluating its relation to the optical chiasma because the tumor may have extra-sellar extension, compressing contiguous structures such as the chiasma itself and the cavernous sinus [1, 9].

The diagnosis of acromegaly, in the average, is usually done with nine years of evolution of the disease - varying from 6.6 to 10.2 years [12]. The establishment of this diagnosis is highly important due to the seriousness of this disease as well as its complications [13]. Patients with acromegaly have approximately a 10-year reduction of expectation of life [14], but 50% of the patients with acromegaly and aged over 50 die due to cardiovascular complications [14]. In patients with acromegaly, cardiovascular disturbances are the cause of death in 24% of the cases, followed by respiratory (18%) and cerebrovascular (14%) disorders [14]. In addition, patients who present high levels of GH have a moderate rise in the risk of appearance of colorectal cancer [15], which can present themselves as more aggressive cancers and develop a rise in the cancer-mortality relation [13, 16]. Conversely, some studies show that patients with acromegaly and GH levels inferior to 2.5 ng/mL have normal life expectancy [1, 17].

The treatment of acromegaly aims to control the growth of the pituitary tumor and the hypersecretion of GH and IGF-1 as well as their long-term effects [10, 18]. A surgical intervention may be carried out through transsphenoidal via for well delimited tumors, displaying excellent results for interventions in microadenomas [19, 20], both for the relief of the compressive effect of the tumoral mass and for the removal of secretory tissue [1]. With surgery, the odds of cure or control of the disease may reach up to 75% [21]. Experienced surgeons can remove maximum tumoral tissue without compromising the physiological function of the adenohypophysis [1, 21]. The tumor may invade the dural space and, even after its resection, continue to secrete [1]. The invasion of the cavernous sinus turns the surgery very dangerous due to the commitment of this neurovascular structure [1]. Besides, a residue of tumoral tissue may remain after the resection which requires a rigorous biochemical control after the surgery [1]. A collateral effect of the surgical treatment is the development of hypopituitarism by excessive resection of the adenohypophysis tissue [22]. As neo-adjuvant or adjuvant measures, radiotherapy [23, 24, 25, 26, 27, 28], dopamine agonists [29], and somatostatin receptor agonists (*Somatotropin release-inhibiting factor* or SRIF) may be used [30, 31]. For the inoperable tumors and for uncontrollable levels of GH and IGF-1 after the surgery, pharmacological schemes with the medications mentioned above may be applicable with the intention of controlling them, where even antagonists of the GH receptor may be used [1]. For improved therapeutic efficiency, these drugs can be combined [32].

GH Deficiency

The GH deficiency (GHD) is a clinical entity characterized by the reduction of the liberation or action of the GH. GH is the most affected hormone in adults when there is some pituitary or hypothalamic deficiency [33] and is invariably reduced when two pituitary hormones are deficient [34]. GHD has a prevalence of 14.5-27/100,000 in the general population [35]. GHD causes deleterious effects in the body, such as the reduction of the fat-free mass, the rise of the fat mass, the rise of cardiovascular diseases with subsequent reduction of the quality of life [36, 37]. Table 2 shows a summary of the effects of the GH deficiency.

Table 2. Effects of GH deficiency

Body composition	Rise in fat mass with alterations in fat distribution, reduction of fat-free mass, rise in the waist-hip ratio
Physical capacity	Reduction of the maximum oxygen capacity, impairment of cardiac function, reduction of muscular mass
Cardiovascular risk factors	Impairment of cardiovascular function and structure, altered lipid profile, reduction of fibrinolytic activity, atherosclerosis, rise in visceral fat, insulin resistance
Radiologic alterations	Mass or other pituitary alterations, bone density reduction, rise in visceral fat
Laboratory data	GH < 3 ng/mL after stimulation, IGF-1 normal or reduced, dyslipidemia, concomitant reduction of gonadotrophins, TSH and/or ACTH.

Adapted from MELMED & KLEINBERG, 2008.

In children, the most common cause of GH deficiency is the idiopathic deficiency, triggered by rare genetic syndromes or abnormalities of the central nervous system [38, 39]. In adults, the GHD is more associated with functioning or non-functioning pituitary tumors that may compress or invade the somatotropes (GH secreting cells) or even as a result of some treatment of these or other intracranial tumors, such as surgery or radiotherapy head and neck [40]. The hypothalamus is more sensitive to radiation than the pituitary gland, which makes the former more frequently affected even with lower doses of radiation [41].

The diagnosis of GHD is based on the GH stimulation test, which can be made with the administration of GHRH and arginine, GHRH and GH liberator peptide (GHRH) or with glucagon [42]. There are three types of stimulation tests due to the existence of specific counter-indications for each type, but only the execution of one test is necessary for the GHD diagnosis. The GHRH + arginine test is the one with higher sensibility and specificity [43]. Nonetheless, not all patients need the GH stimulation test for the diagnosis of GHD [43]. If the patient has deficiency of three or more pituitary hormones and reduction of the IGF-1 level, there is more than 97% of possibility of this patient having GH deficiency [43].

There are three conditions where the GH stimulation test is necessary: (1) in patients with signs and symptoms of hypothalamic-pituitary deficiency, whether of endocrinologic, structural, or genetic origin; (2) in patients that suffered radiation in head or neck areas or intra-cranial tumors treatment and

(3) in patients that suffered cranial-encephalic traumatism (CET) or subdural hematomas [43].

The cutting points for diagnosis through each GH stimulation test are different, where the ones of the tests with GHRH and GHRP and with glucagon a GH peak inferior to 3 ng/mL [43, 44, 45]. GH's response to the GHRH and arginine test is related to the body mass index (BMI) of the patients, where the cutting point for patients with BMI inferior to 25 kg/m² is a peak inferior to 11 ng/mL, while for those with BMI between 25 and 30 kg/m², the peak would be inferior to 8 ng/mL; for BMI superior to 30 kg/m², a peak inferior to 4 ng/mL [43].

The aim of the treatment of GHD is to correct the metabolic, functional, and psychological deficiencies [43]. Every patient when diagnosed with GHD receives a recommendation to carry out the treatment through the GH replacement [43]. The objective of the replacement is to promote its benefits without causing collateral effects [43]. By the studies carried out, we know that younger people have more GH secretion than older people, and women more than men; as a result, we start the treatment with doses of 0.3 mg/day in young people, 0.2 mg/day in women, and 0.1mg/day in older people. The adjustment of the dose according to weight is not recommended due to the great difference of sensibility of each individual [43].

The replacement must be made at night preferably, with the intent to mimic the normal cycle of GH liberation, which has its peak during this phase of the day. The dose must be individually adjusted with the ongoing organic answers to the respective doses [43].

Quality of Life in Acromegaly and GH Deficiency

The quality of life (QoL) of any person, whether in the physical, social, emotional, or psychological fields will be impaired by the existence of any health problem [46]. Nevertheless, the difficulty resides in quantifying how much a determined disease affects the quality of life of the patients [47, 48].

Acromegaly

Acromegaly is a disease with significant reduction of QoL demonstrated by diverse questionnaires, whether specific or generic [46, 47, 48, 49]. Between the many clinical manifestations and comorbidities present in acromegaly, the ones that mostly compromise QoL are pain, body self-image, emotional lability, depression, strength and energy reduction [46].

According to the study of Webb et al. (2006), there are some factors that demonstrate a worse QoL associated with acromegaly: active disease, feminine gender, age, length of disease, presence of joint symptoms, and previous radiotherapy. The study of Kauppinen-Makelin et al. (2006), as well as the one by Webb et al. (2006), demonstrated a better QoL in younger patients, with lower BMI, and who did not receive previous radiotherapy. Despite that, contrary to Webb's study, this study affirms that there is no influence of the patient's gender on QoL, in addition to not demonstrating significant association of the latter with the surgical treatment of acromegaly, GH concentration at the moment of diagnosis, use of medication to reduce the GH levels, or the presence of hypopituitarism, hypertension, or Diabetes Mellitus. There are many non-specific questionnaires that can and have already been used to quantify the QoL in patients with acromegaly, such as the *Short-Form Health Survey* (SF-36) [46], the *Signs and Symptoms Scores* (SSS), the *Psychological General Wellbeing Schedule* (PGWBS), and the EuroQoL (EQ 5-D) [47], but in 2002, with the work of Webb, we were granted with an important tool, the AcroQoL. This is a questionnaire specific to measure the QoL in patients with acromegaly [46, 47, 49]. The questionnaire was developed in Spain and considers physical, psychological, and social aspects, daily activities, symptoms, cognition, general health, sleep, sexual function, pain, energy, and body image [46, 49].

According to Trepp et al. (2005), the patients with acromegaly whose GH and IGF-1 biochemical levels are elevated have a worse quality of life when compared to patients with well controlled biochemical levels. The items of AcroQoL (Table 3) that demonstrate with more clarity the differences in the QoL between patients with controlled and uncontrolled biochemical levels were the items 2 (*I feel ugly*), 5 (*I avoid going out very much with friends because of my appearance),* 8 (*I feel rejected by people because of my illness),* 9 *(I have problems carrying out my usual activities),* 13 (*The illness affects my performance at work or in my usual tasks),* 19 (*I feel like a sick person),* and 20 (*The physical changes produced by my illness govern my life),* demonstrating to be the best to evaluate the remission or persistence of the disease [49]. Even with a rigorous control and adequate treatment of the acromegaly, many patients present, after treatment, a reduced QoL owed to the many definitive manifestations that the excess of GH and IGF-1 cause on the body of the patients. Some treatments are also related to the reduction of QoL in patients with a controlled disease [52].

There are many therapeutic modalities for the control of the acromegaly. These can be surgical, pharmacotherapy, or radiotherapy, or even an association of them. The technological advances in all these therapeutic modalities permit the cure of virtually all the patients [48, 52]. The expectations are that, with the progress of these technological advances, we will be able to go beyond the control of biochemical parameters and also control the other aspects inherent to the acromegaly, such as the visual alterations, the size of pituitary adenoma, alterations of the soft tissues, and most of all, the quality of life of the patients [48].

Table 3. Questionnaire ACROQOL

1	My legs feel weak
2	I feel ugly
3	I get depressed
4	I look awful in photographs
5	I avoid going out very much with friends because of my appearance
6	I try to avoid socializing
7	I look different in the mirror
8	I feel rejected by people because of my illness
9	I have problems carrying out my usual activities
10	People stare at me because of my appearance
11	Some parts of my body (nose, feet, hands,...) are too big
12	I have problems doing things with my hands, e.g. sewing or handling tools
13	The illness affects my performance at work or in my usual tasks
14	My joints ache
15	I am usually tired
16	I snore at night
17	It is hard for me to articulate words due to the size of my tongue
18	I have problems with sexual relationships
19	I feel like a sick person
20	The physical changes produced by my illness govern my life
21	I have little sexual appetite
22	I fell weak

The frequency of occurrence (always, most of the time, sometimes, rarely, never) or the degree of agreement with the item (completely agree, moderately agree, neither agree nor disagree, moderately disagree, completely disagree). Those are the answers.

Adapted from TREPP et al., 2005.

There are few studies demonstrating the improvement of QoL in relation to the diverse types of treatment [47]. The use of lanreotide, 30 mg every 14 days, during 2 months, in patients with active acromegaly demonstrated a significant reduction on the GH and IGF-1 levels and also showed an improvement in the QoL of these patients [53]. There seems to be a real relation between the IGF-1 levels and the scores on the AcroQoL, a relation that is not observed on the non-specific questionnaires, SSS, PGWBS and the EQ 5-D [47].

The study of Van der Klaauw et al. (2008) compared patients who received isolated surgical treatment to those that received radiotherapy treatment after the surgery and to others who received treatment with somatostatin analogues. This study demonstrated that the patients who received radiotherapy after surgery, compared to the ones who only received surgical treatment, evolved with a reduction of the physical function, more pain, and greater loss of energy.

There is still divergence about the relation of the IGF-1 levels and the QoL of the patients. According to the study of Rowles et al. (2005), there is no relation between its levels and QoL. The study of Paisley et al. (2007) concluded the contrary, claiming the existence of connection between the reduction of the IGF-1 levels and the improvement of QoL, and it states that this correlation is more evident in patients with the active disease than those in remission.

GH Deficiency

The QoL of patients with GHD is lower than that of control groups. The reduction of the QoL in GHD seems to be related to the reduction of energy and the decrease of physical activity, in addition to psycho-emotional problems, such as the reduction of concentration and social isolation due to psychological suffering [54, 55, 56]. Besides, patients with GHD seem to have a reduction in sleep quality because GH and GHRH are closely connected to the sleep physiology and are altered in the GHD. This reduction of the sleep quality seems to be one of the main causes of diurnal fatigue, which is one of the most frequent complaints and one of the main causes of the reduction of QoL in patients with GHD [57].

The study of QoL in patients with GHD has used non-specific questionnaires, such as the PGWBS, the SF-36, and the *Nottingham Health Profile* (NHP) as tools that, just like in the acromegaly, are little sensitive to specific alterations of the diseases studied. Nonetheless, they are excellent tools when used to compare the QoL in different diseases [54, 55]. Specifically designed for patients with GHD, the *QOL-Assessment of Growth Hormone Deficiency in Adults* (QoL-AGHDA) was developed with the intention of evaluating with more accuracy all the effects of GHD and their relations to QoL, and estimating the benefits of the GH replacement therapy [55].

Table 4. Questions on Life Satisfaction - Hypopituitarism

How important for you is (are) your...	Not Important	Somewhat Important	Important	Very Important	Extremely important
Resilience/ability to tolerate stress					
Body Shape					
Self confidence					
Ability to become sexually aroused					
Concentration					
Physical stamina					
Initiative/drive					
Ability to cope with your own anger					
Ability to tolerate noise and disturbance					
How satisfied are you with your…	Dissatisfied	Somewhat Dissatisfied	Somewhat Satisfied	Satisfied	Very Satisfied
Resilience/ability to tolerate stress					
Body Shape					
Self confidence					
Ability to become sexually aroused					
Concentration					
Physical stamina					
Initiative/drive					
Ability to cope with your own anger					
Resilience/ability to tolerate stress					

Adapted from HERSCHBACH et al., 2001.

In 2001, Herschbach et al. developed another specific questionnaire, the QLS^{M}-H (*Questions on Life Satisfaction Modules*) (Table 4). This questionnaire was developed due to the necessity of evaluating with more accuracy the QoL in patients with hypopituitarism. A second objective was taken into account for the elaboration of this questionnaire: the necessity of evaluating more efficiently the QoL internationally, in the different cultural situations, allowing the comparison of data from different points of the globe with more security and reliability. Its developers implemented questions in the beginning of the referred questionnaire about the importance of each item. As a result, this kind of instrument takes into account whether determined answers have considerable importance or not in the life of that person [58, 59].

According to the study of Koltowska-Häggström et al. (2008), women with GHD have worse QoL than men in the same condition, before treatment. The greater gain in QoL happened during the first year of treatment, although, from this point on, no significant difference between men and women is observed. The same study also established a relation between the reduction of the QoL and the age progression. In addition, it demonstrated that patients who developed GHD as a result of pituitary adenoma had a worse QoL than the patients with GHD resulting from other causes. These lower scores in the QoL occurred both before and after the treatment. Nevertheless, the cause of GHD did not demonstrate having influence on the response to treatment neither on the total nor the annual gain of QoL. Previous treatments, such as surgery or radiotherapy also did not exert influence over the QoL or the response to treatment with GH [60].

Patients who developed GHD during childhood have better QoL than patients who developed it during adulthood, both before and after the treatment. Nevertheless, patients who developed GHD during childhood have a lower gain in total and annual QoL with the GH replacement than the patients who presented GHD during adult life [60].

Patients with GHD since childhood, even when receiving GH replacement treatment, presented during adult life higher levels of unemployment or insertion in less valued jobs, a social difficulty that promotes even lower marriage rates for the patients in relation to the general population. Allied to this, there is also a reduction of the general health perception [61].

The study of Attanasio et al. (2005) demonstrated a severe reduction of the QoL in young patients that developed the GHD in childhood. Nonetheless, the same study revealed that patients affected by the GHD in childhood presented a better response of QoL to GH replacement than those affected in adulthood. Even with the results of this study, it is not clear yet whether the reduction of QoL in adult patients with GHD developed during the childhood would be more related to the consequences deriving of the GHD in childhood, in the adult life, or an association of its effects throughout the life of the patient.

Patients with a deficiency of multiple pituitary hormones did not present a worse QoL than those with isolated GHD. In addition, the response of QoL to GH replacement therapy was similar in patients with multiple hormone deficiency and those with isolated GHD [60].

Patients with GHD and comorbidities have a significant reduction of the QoL. Despite this, after the treatment with GH, these patients have a total and annual gain in QoL higher than the patients without comorbidities [60].

Since the commercial availability of the recombining GH, the treatment with GH replacement (GHR) on high doses was instituted with excellent results, however, there are collateral effects, such as hydric retention and arthralgia, which may be responsible for the abandonment of treatment. There are still more severe potential collateral effects, such as the increase of incidence of breast and prostate cancers [55].

After the use of GHR, the majority of the studies demonstrated a significant increase in the QoL, in addition to the improvement on the lipid profile, with a reduction of the total cholesterol and LDL cholesterol. Furthermore, the GHR promotes reduction of fat mass and rise of lean mass [54, 55].

The use of low doses of GHR with the aim of reaching physiological levels of IGF-1 resulted in an improvement of the QoL within just one month of treatment, with an even greater improvement within three months of treatment. It is important to mention that the GHR in low doses also provided an improvement of physical aspects, such as the reduction of fat mass, rise of lean mass, and the reduction of waist-hip relation [55].

Final Considerations

These studies demonstrated that the sooner the treatment of the acromegaly and the GHD are implemented, the better the QoL of these patients will be. Despite this, these treatments must be properly suggested, controlled, and followed, because in there are diverse collateral effects that may reduce considerably the QoL of the patients in both diseases.

References

[1] Melmed S., Kleinberg D. Anterior Pituitary. KRONENBERG H. M. et al. In: *Williams textbook of endocrinology*, 11. ed. Philadelphia, USA: Saunders Elsevier; 2008, 155-262.

[2] Barinaga M., Yamonoto G., Rivier C., Vale W., Evans R., Rosenfeld M. G. Transcriptional regulation of growth hormone gene expression by growth hormone-releasing factor. *Nature*, 1983, 306(5938):84-85.

[3] Thorner M. O., Frohman L. A., Leong D. A., Thominet J., Downs T., Hellmann P. et al. Extrahypothalamic growth-hormone-releasing factor (GRF) secretion is a rare cause of acromegaly: plasma GRF levels in 177 acromegalic patients. *J Clin Endocrinol Metab,* 1984, 59(5):846-849.

[4] Van Cauter E., Plat L., Copinschi G. Interrelations between sleep and the somatotropic axis. *Sleep,* 1998, 21(6):553-566.

[5] Feinberg I. Slow wave sleep and release of growth hormone. *JAMA*. 2000, 284(21):2717-8.

[6] Ho K. Y., Veldhuis J. D., Johnson M. L., Furlanetto R., Evans W. S., Alberti K. G. et al. Fasting enhances growth hormone secretion and amplifies the complex rhythms of growth hormone secretion in man. *J Clin Invest.,* 1988, 81(4):968-975.

[7] Vigneri R., Squatrito S., Pezzino V., Filetti S., Branca S., Polosa P. Growth hormone levels in diabetes. Correlation with the clinical control of the disease. *Diabetes,* 1976, 25(3):167-172.

[8] Ben-Shlomo A., Melmed S. Acromegaly. *Endocrinol Metab Clin North Am.,* 2008, 37(1):101-122.

[9] Melmed S. Acromegaly: Melmed S. *The pituitary*. Cambridge, USA: Blackwell; 1995, 413-442.

[10] Giustina A., Barkan A., Casanueva F. F., Cavagnini F., Frohman L., Ho K. et al. Criteria for cure of acromegaly: a consensus statement. *J Clin Endocrinol Metab.,* 2000, 85(2):526-529.

[11] Duncan E., Was J. A. Investigation protocol: acromegaly and its investigation. *Clin Endocrinol.,* 1999, 50(3):285-293.

[12] Jadresic A., Banks L. M., Child D. F., Diamant L., Doyle F. H., Fraser T. R. et al. The acromegaly syndrome. Relation between clinical features, growth hormone values and radiological characteristics of the pituitary tumours. *Q J Med.,* 1982, 51(202):189-204.

[13] Giustina A., Casanueva F. F., Cavagnini F., Chanson P., Clemmons D., Frohman L. A. et al. Diagnosis and treatment of acromegaly complications. *J Endocrinol Invest.,* 2003, 26(12):1242-1247.

[14] Rajasoorya C., Holdaway I. M., Wrightson P., Scott D. J., Ibbertson H. K. Determinants of clinical outcome and survival in acromegaly. *Clin Endocrinol.,* 1994, 41(1):95-102.

[15] Renehan A. G., O'Connell J., O'Halloran D., Shanahan F., Potten C. S., O'Dwyer S. T. et al. Acromegaly and colorectal cancer: a comprehensive review of epidemiology, biological mechanisms, and clinical implications. *Horm Metab Res.,* 2003, 35:712-725.

[16] Orme S. M., McNally R. J., Cartwright R. A., Belchetz P. E. Mortality and cancer incidence in acromegaly: a retrospective cohort study. United Kingdom Acromegaly Study Group. *J Clin Endocrinol Metab.,* 1998, 83(8):2730-2734.

[17] Bates A. S., Van't Hoff W., Jones J. M., Clayton R. N. An audit of outcome of treatment in acromegaly. *Q J Med.,* 1993, 86(5):293-299.

[18] Melmed S., Jackson I., Kleinberg D., Klibanski A. Current treatment guidelines for acromegaly. *J Clin Endocrinol Metab.,* 1998, 83(8):2646-2652.

[19] Lissett C. A., Peacey S. R., Laing I., Tetlow L., Davis J. R., Shalet S. M. The outcome of surgery for acromegaly: the need for a specialist pituitary surgeon for all types of growth hormone (GH) secreting adenoma. *Clin Endocrinol.,* 1998, 49(5):653-657.

[20] Fahlbusch R., Keller B., Ganslandt O., Kreutzer J., Nimsky C. Transsphenoidal surgery in acromegaly investigated by intraoperative high-field magnetic resonance imaging. *Eur J Endocrinol.,* 2005, 153(2):239-248.

[21] Madsen M., Poulsen P. L., Orskov H., Møller N.,; Jørgensen J. O. Cotreatment with pegvisomant and a somatostatin analog (SA) in SA-responsive acromegalic patients. *J Clin Endocrinol Metab.,* 2011, 96(8):2405-2413.

[22] Kreutzer J., Vance M. L., Lopes M. B., Laws Jr E. R. Surgical management of GH-secreting pituitary adenomas: an outcome study using modern remission criteria. *J Clin Endocrinol Metab.,* 2001, 86(9):4072-4077.

[23] Barrande G., Pittino-Lungo M., Coste J., Ponvert D., Bertagna X., Luton J. P. et al. Hormonal and metabolic effects of radiotherapy in acromegaly: long-term results in 128 patients followed in a single center. *J Clin Endocrinol Metab.,* 2000, 85(10):3779-3785.

[24] Biermasz N. R., van Dulken H., Roelfsema F. Long-term follow-up results of postoperative radiotherapy in 36 patients with acromegaly. *J Clin Endocrinol Metab.,* 2000, 85(7):2476-2482.

[25] Eastman R. C., Gorden P., Glatstein E., Roth J. Radiation therapy of acromegaly. *Endocrinol Metab Clin North Am.,* 1992, 21(3):693-712.

[26] Barkan A. L., Halasz I., Dornfeld K. J., Jaffe C. A., Friberg R. D., Chandler W. F. et al. Pituitary irradiation is ineffective in normalizing plasma insulin-like growth factor I in patients with acromegaly. *J Clin Endocrinol Metab.,* 1997, 82(10):3187-3191.

[27] Powell J. S., Wardlaw S. L., Post K. D., Freda P. U. Outcome of radiotherapy for acromegaly using normalization of insulin-like growth factor I to define cure. *J Clin Endocrinol Metab.,* 2000, 85(5):2068-2071.

[28] Jezková J., Marek J., Hána V., Krsek M., Weiss V., Vladyka V. et al. Gamma knife radiosurgery for acromegaly--long-term experience. *Clin Endocrinol.,* 2006, 64(5):588-595.

[29] Colao A., Ferone D., Cappabianca P., del Basso De Caro M. L., Marzullo P., Monticelli A. et al. Effect of octreotide pretreatment on surgical outcome in acromegaly. *J Clin Endocrinol Metab.,* 1997, 82(10):3308-3314.

[30] Colao A., Di Sarno A., Sarnacchiaro F., Ferone D., Di Renzo G., Merola B. et al. Prolactinomas resistant to standard dopamine agonists respond to chronic cabergoline treatment. *J Clin Endocrinol Metab.,* 1997, 82(3):876-883.

[31] Biermasz N. R., van Dulken H., Roelfsema F. Direct postoperative and follow-up results of transsphenoidal surgery in 19 acromegalic patients pretreated with octreotide compared to those in untreated matched controls. *J Clin Endocrinol Metab.,* 1999, 84(10):3551-3555.

[32] Jørgensen J. O., Feldt-Rasmussen U., Frystyk J., Chen J. W., Kristensen L. Ø., Hagen C. et al. Cotreatment of acromegaly with a somatostatin analog and a growth hormone receptor antagonist. *J Clin Endocrinol Metab.,* 2005, 90(10):5627-5631.

[33] *Abs R.,* Bengtsson B. A., Hernberg-Stâhl E., Monson J. P., Tauber J. P., Wilton P. et al. GH Replacement in 1034 Growth Hormone Deficient Hypopituitary Adults: Demographic and Clinical Characteristics, Dosing and Safety. *Clin Endocrinol.,* 1999, 50(6):703-713.

[34] Drake W. M., Howell S. J., Monson J.P., Shalet S. M. Optimizing GH therapy in adults and children. *Endocr Rev.,* 2001, 22(4):425-450.

[35] Vimpani G. V., Vimpani A. F., Lidgard G. P. Cameron, EH; Farquhar, JW. Prevalence of severe growth hormone deficiency. *Br Med J.,* 1977, 2(6084):427-430.

[36] de Boer H., Blok G. J., Van der Veen E. A. Clinical aspects of growth hormone deficiency in adults. *Endocr Rev.,* 1995, 16(1):63-86.

[37] Molitch M. E., Clemmons D. R., Malozowski S., Merriam G. R., Shalet S. M., Vance M. L. et al. Evaluation and treatment of adult growth hormone deficiency: an Endocrine Society Clinical Practice Guideline. *J Clin Endocrinol Metab.,* 2006, 91(5):1621-1634.

[38] Allen D. B., Fost N. C. Growth hormone therapy for short stature: panacea or Pandora's box? *J Pediatr.,* 1990, 117(1 Pt 1):16-21.

[39] Clayton P. E., Price D. A., Shalet S. M. Growth hormone state after completion of treatment with growth hormone. *Arch Dis Child.,* 1987, 62(3):222-6.

[40] Schmiegelow M., Lassen S., Poulsen H. S., Feldt-Rasmussen U., Schmiegelow K., Hertz H. et al. Cranial radiotherapy of childhood brain tumours: growth hormone deficiency and its relation to the biological effective dose of irradiation in a large population based study. *Clin Endocrinol.,* 2000, 53(2):191-197.

[41] Sklar C. A., Constine L. S. Chronic neuroendocrinological sequelae of radiation therapy. *Int J Radiat Oncol Biol Phys.,* 1995, 31(5):1113-1121.

[42] Reiter E. O., Rosenfifeld R. G. Normal and Aberrant Growth. Kronenberg H. M. et al. In: *Williams textbook of endocrinology*, 11. ed. Philadelphia, USA: Saunders Elsevier; 2008, 849-941.

[43] Ho K. K. 2007 GH Deficiency Consensus Workshop Participants. Consensus guidelines for the diagnosis and treatment of adults with GH deficiency II: a statement of the GH Research Society in association with the European Society for Pediatric Endocrinology, Lawson Wilkins Society, European Society of Endocrinology, Japan Endocrine Society, and Endocrine Society of Australia. *Eur J Endocrinol.,* 2007, 157(6):695-700.

[44] Consensus guidelines for the diagnosis and treatment of adults with growth hormone deficiency: summary statement of the Growth Hormone Research Society Workshop on Adult Growth Hormone Deficiency. *J Clin Endocrinol Metab.,* 1998, 83(2):379-81.

[45] Carroll, PV; Christ, ER; Bengtsson, BA; Carlsson, L; Christiansen, JS; Clemmons, D et al. Growth hormone deficiency in adulthood and the effects of growth hormone replacement: a review. Growth Hormone

Research Society Scientific Committee. *J Clin Endocrinol Metab.,* 1998 Feb;83(2):382-95.

[46] Webb S. M., Prieto L., Badia X., Albareda M., Catalá M., Gaztambide S. et al. Acromegaly Quality of Life Questionnaire (ACROQOL) a new health-related quality of life questionnaire for patients with acromegaly: development and psychometric properties. *Clin Endocrinol.,* 2002, 57(2):251-8.

[47] Paisley A. N., Rowles S. V., Roberts M. E., Webb S. M., Badia X., Prieto L. et al. Treatment of acromegaly improves quality of life, measured by AcroQol. *Clin Endocrinol.,* 2007, 67(3):358-362.

[48] Rowles S. V., Prieto L., Badia X., Shalet S. M., Webb S. M., Trainer P. J. Quality of life (QOL) in patients with acromegaly is severely impaired: use of a novel measure of QOL: acromegaly quality of life questionnaire. *J Clin Endocrinol Metab.,* 2005, 90(6):3337-3341.

[49] Trepp R., Everts R., Stettler C., Fischli S., Allemann S., Webb S. M. et al. Assessment of quality of life in patients with uncontrolled vs. controlled acromegaly using the Acromegaly Quality of Life Questionnaire (AcroQoL). *Clin Endocrinol.,* 2005, 63(1):103-110.

[50] Webb S. M. Quality of life in acromegaly. *Neuroendocrinology,* 2006, 83(3-4):224-229.

[51] Kauppinen-Mäkelin R., Sane T., Sintonen H., Markkanen H., Välimäki M. J., Löyttyniemi E. et al. Quality of life in treated patients with acromegaly. *J Clin Endocrinol Metab.,* 2006, 91(10):3891-3896.

[52] van der Klaauw A. A., Biermasz N. R., Hoftijzer H. C., Pereira A. M., Romijn J. A. Previous radiotherapy negatively influences quality of life during 4 years of follow-up in patients cured from acromegaly. *Clin Endocrinol.,* 2008, 69(1):123-128.

[53] Sonino, N; Scarpa, E; Paoletta, A; Fallo, F; Boscaro, M. Slow-release lanreotide treatment in acromegaly: effects on quality of life. *Psychother Psychosom.* 1999;68(3):165-167.

[54] Li Voon Chong J. S., Benbow S., Foy P., Wallymahmed M. E., Wile D., MacFarlane I. A. Elderly people with hypothalamic-pituitary disease and growth hormone deficiency: lipid profiles, body composition and quality of life compared with control subjects. *Clin Endocrinol.,* 2000, 53(5):551-559.

[55] Ahmad AM., Hopkins M. T., Thomas J., Ibrahim H., Fraser W. D., Vora J. P. Body composition and quality of life in adults with growth hormone deficiency; effects of low-dose growth hormone replacement. *Clin Endocrinol.,* 2001, 54(6):709-717.

[56] Gilchrist F. J., Murray R. D., Shalet S. M. The effect of long-term untreated growth hormone deficiency (GHD) and 9 years of GH replacement on the quality of life (QoL) of GH-deficient adults. *Clin Endocrinol.,* 2002, 57(3):363-370.

[57] Copinschi G., Nedeltcheva A., Leproult R., Morselli L. L., Spiegel, K; Martino, E et al. Sleep disturbances, daytime sleepiness, and quality of life in adults with growth hormone deficiency. *J Clin Endocrinol Metab.* 2010 May;95(5):2195-2202.

[58] Herschbach P., Henrich G., Strasburger C. J., Feldmeier H., Marín F., Attanasio A. M. et al. Development and psychometric properties of a disease-specific quality of life questionnaire for adult patients with growth hormone deficiency. *Eur J Endocrinol.,* 2001, 145(3):255-265.

[59] Rosilio M., Blum W. F., Edwards D. J., Shavrikova E. P., Valle D., Lamberts S. W. et al. Long-term improvement of quality of life during growth hormone (GH) replacement therapy in adults with GH deficiency, as measured by questions on life satisfaction-hypopituitarism (QLS-H). *J Clin Endocrinol Metab.,* 2004, 89(4):1684-1693.

[60] Kołtowska-Häggström M., Kind P., Monson J. P., Jonsson B. Growth hormone (GH) replacement in hypopituitary adults with GH deficiency evaluated by a utility-weighted quality of life index: a precursor to cost-utility analysis. *Clin Endocrinol.,* 2008, 68(1):122-129.

[61] Attanasio A. F., Shavrikova E. P., Blum W. F., Shalet S. M. Quality of life in childhood onset growth hormone-deficient patients in the transition phase from childhood to adulthood. *J Clin Endocrinol Metab.,* 2005, 90(8):4525-4529.

In: Quality of Life in Endocrine Diseases ISBN: 978-1-63463-911-8
Editor: Erika Cesar de Oliveira Naliato © 2015 Nova Science Publishers, Inc.

Chapter 5

Quality of Life and Cushing's Syndrome*

Vanessa T. O. Rezende, Thiago R. Ferreira and Erika C. O. Naliato*

Center of Studies Ricardo A. T. Castilho of the Teresópolis Medical Association, Brazil

Abbreviations

BMD	bone mineral density
CD	Cushing's disease
CS	Cushing's Syndrome
CT	computerized tomography
DM2	diabetes mellitus type 2
HRQL	Health-Related Quality of Life
NHP	Nottingham Health Profile
SAH	systemic arterial hypertension
SCS	subclinical Cushing's Syndrome
SF-36	Short Health Evaluation Form 36

* Correspondence to: erikanaliato@uol.com.br.

Introduction

Cushing's syndrome (CS) is a condition caused by the exposure, of long term, to high levels of glucocorticoids, endogenous or exogenous [1, 2]. The CS may be divided into two groups: ACTH-dependent and ACTH-independent [3, 4]. The ACTH-dependent CS occurs by the rise in the liberation of ACTH, due to a pituitary adenoma, an increase in the secretion of the corticotrophin release hormone (CRH), an ectopic liberation, [2,5] or an uncertain ACTH source [3]. The ACTH-independent CS, in 20% to 30% of the cases is due to primary adrenal lesions. The cortisol producing adenomas and carcinomas - usually unilateral - are frequently easily visualized in a CT scan. Other causes of adrenal lesions are bilateral primary pigmented nodular hyperplasia, macronodular adrenal hyperplasia, aberrant expression of hormone receptors in adrenal cortex, McCune–Albright syndrome and Carney complex [5].

Causes

The most common cause of CS is the chronic use of glucocorticoids (exogenous) [3] whether orally administered, inhalant, or even topic [5, 6]. The risk of exogenous CS (ECS) is increased when there is an association of glucocorticoids with medicines that inhibit the cytochrome P450 [6].

Rare cases of CS include the adenomatous transformation of the ectopic adrenal tissue, cortisol-secreting ovarian tumors and even the remains of adrenal cells, located on the testicles, producing cortisol [5, 7, 8].

A very rare cause of ACTH-dependent CS is the ectopic expression of hormonal receptors on the adrenal cortex [9, 10].

The ectopic ACTH syndrome is caused by bronchial carcinoids tumors, medullary thyroid carcinomas and prostatic carcinomas [11, 12]. It is rarer than the isolated secretion of CRH [2].

The most common cause of endogenous CS is the ACTH-secreting pituitary adenoma [13]. The CS caused by ACTH-secreting pituitary tumors is named Cushing's Disease (CD) [2, 5, 4] and it leads to bilateral adrenal hyperplasia or macronodular hyperplasia [3]. CD is more prevalent in the feminine gender in a 8:1 proportion. In general, it starts between 20 and 40 years of age and has a slow progression [3].

Many of its clinical-laboratory manifestations are observed in more frequent diseases [3, 5].

Clinical Manifestations

The CS clinical state involves signs of general, skin, musculoskeletal, neuropsychiatric, gonadal, and metabolic symptoms. They are: weight gain/obesity, weakness, arterial hypertension, moon *facies*, edema, "buffalo hump", female baldness, electrocardiographic abnormalities, atherosclerosis, skin thinning, hirsutism, plethora, stretch marks, facial contusions, acne, diminished cicatrization, osteopenia, fracture, depression, emotional lability, headache, menstrual alterations, reduction of libido, erectile dysfunction, glucose intolerance, dyslipidemia, polyuria, nephrolithiasis and hypokalemic alkalosis [13].

Due to the antagonism of cortisol and IGF-1 in the growth plate, the CS leads to important reduction of children's growth [14, 15].

Patients with subclinical CS (SCS) have a high prevalence of obesity, systemic arterial hypertension (SAH), diabetes mellitus type 2 (DM2), in addition to rise of the bone turnover and the reduction of bone mineral density (BMD) [16, 17]. The SCS is a result of a silent adrenal adenoma and rarely evolves to the classic form of CS.

Diagnosis

The diagnosis of CS may be difficult in some cases of ACTH-dependent CS, where the cortisol secretion as well as the signs and symptoms of the syndrome are cyclical [5, 18, 19].

By excluding the exogenous hypercortisolism, the CS investigation comprehends the confirmation of hypercortisolism – by the low-dose dexametasone suppression test (which evaluates whether the administration of low doses of dexametasone is able to inhibit the ACTH and, as a result, the cortisol, as it occurs in the normal individual) [20-21], through the urinary free cortisol measurements (from a 24-hour urine sample) [3, 20], the evaluation of the serum cortisol level at midnight (period when, in the normal cortisol circadian cycle, the serum and cortisol levels are lower, but they get higher in the CS) [2, 20, 21] and the evaluation of the saliva cortisol level by the end of the night (correlating withe the levels of plasma free cortisol) [22, 23].

Treatment

Without treatment, 50% of the patients die in 5 years [13]. The treatment of CS depends on its etiology.

The exogenous CS is solved by the gradual reduction of exogenous glucocorticoids.

In the cases of CD, transsphenoidal adenomectomy may be conducted, with the benefit of being a fast cure treatment that does not lead to other significant hormonal alterations (or transcranial adenomectomy, for larger tumors); it is also possible to opt for radiotherapy (usually when surgery is not successful, and associated with an anti-adrenal agent to accelerate the drop of cortisol levels) or a pharmacological treatment (indicated in preoperative period, associated with radiotherapy or in etiology unknown ACTH-dependents) The available drugs are inhibitors of the adrenal steroidogenesis - where the ketoconazole is the most frequently used - the neuromodulators of ACTH secretion and the cortisol antagonists [2, 24, 25, 26, 27, 28].

Another treatment option is bilateral adrenalectomy, reserved to persistent, relapsing cases or to aggressive cases of unknown etiology ACTH-dependent CS [24, 29].

The ectopic ACTH syndrome, resulting from the liberation of ACTH by neoplasia, carcinoid or occult tumors has its therapeutic basis on the treatment of neoplasia (such as surgery or chemotherapy) and of hypercortisolism (with hypocortisolemic drugs or adrenalectomy - in the case of non-localized or undetected tumors) [24, 27, 30-37].

In cases of adrenal etiology, unilateral adrenalectomy is performed with therapeutic success although the recovery of the hypothalamus-pituitary-adrenal axis takes longer [38, 39]. Bilateral adrenalectomy, in the case of benign tumors, is the treatment of choice, despite that it presents high morbidity. However, when caused by adrenal carcinomas, there are already metastases by the time of diagnosis [40-42].

In general, the treatment is performed through surgery (ideal for small tumors and those without metastases), radiotherapy (for locally or distant advanced tumors) and drug therapy (controlling the cortisol secretion and, in a lesser degree, inducing volumetric tumor reduction - minotane is the drug of choice) [27, 38, 43].

When resulting from alterations in adrenal cells receptors (non ACTH-dependent CS), CS may be treated with octreotide (if dependent of inhibitory-gastric peptide), propranolol (if adrenal is stimulated by catecholamines), or leuprolide (when LH dependent) [44, 45].

Gómez et al. (2007) [46] investigated the persistence of arterial hypertension in patients with Cushing's treated with ketoconazole and surgery and noted the benefit in the use of ketoconazole, independently of the cause of the CS, since there has been a significant remission of arterial hypertension. Many patients not treated with this scheme remain hypertensive even with the normalization of the glucocorticoids levels. Despite that, some factors, such as advanced age, longer duration of disease, and family history of arterial hypertension, presented negative influence on the remission of hypertension.

Quality of Life

Questionnaires for the Evaluation of QoL in Cushing's Syndrome

There are no specific questionnaires to evaluate quality of life (QoL) in patients with CS; as a result, unspecific questionnaires are used.

The Short Health Evaluation Form 36 (Short Form 36 – SF-36) is a questionnaire that evaluates the following aspects of health: physical functionality, social activities limitations due to physical or emotional problems, limitations in usual activities due to the disease, body pain, general mental health state, limitation of usual activities due to emotional problems, vitality (energy and fatigue), and general mental health - formed by 36 questions with scores of 0 to 100 for each category.

It is an unspecific questionnaire, which allows the comparison of QoL in many diseases and the evaluation of the answer to treatment. It is considered the best generic questionnaire for QoL evaluation [47-52].

The Nottingham Health Profile (NHP) is a self-administered questionnaire very popular for the evaluation of quality of life in patients with pituitary diseases (it was developed to evaluate the QoL in patients with chronic diseases), formed by 38 questions (which answers are "yes" or "no") that evaluate incapacities, such as pain, level of energy, sleep, emotional reactions, social isolation and physical skills, with scores from 0 to 100 for each scale of incapacity. Higher scores are related to worse QoL. Despite informing physical, social, and emotional health, it does not measure all the QoL domains and scores only two levels of skill [53-56].

The Multidimensional Fatigue Inventory (MFI-20) evaluates fatigue in different dimensions: general fatigue, physical fatigue, reduction of activity, reduction of motivation, and mental fatigue. The higher the scores (which vary from 0 to 20), the higher the fatigue level is [57, 58].

The Hospital Anxiety and Depression Scale evaluates the anxiety and depression in sick and healthy people with a scoring for each subscale of 0-21 (total of 0 to 42) - without interference of somatic disturbance in its score. The higher the score, the most serious the symptoms of anxiety and depression are. The application of the scale is fast and simple which can be done by an interviewer or patients themselves [59].

Hypercortisolism and Quality of Life

The Health-Related Quality of Life (HRQL) of patients with CS is compromised by physical and psychological symptoms [60, 61]. The CS leads to obesity, hypertension, insulin resistance, coagulopathy, metabolic syndrome, bone problems, nephrolithiasis, kidney insufficiency, hypothyroidism, hypogonadism, bone mass reduction, osteoarthritis, mental and behavior disturbances, immunosuppression, and cerebral atrophy [62]. All these complications may incur in an impairment of the QoL of individuals with CS [63].

Johnson et al. (2003) [64] developed a research using the SF-36 to patients with adenoma/pituitary hyper-secretion, among which there were the following diseases: CS, acromegaly, prolactinoma and non-functioning macroadenoma, where the questionnaire results were compared between the different groups and those with the normal population (average score of 50 for each category). The scores of patients with CS were significantly lower than those of the general population and of the patients with other types of pituitary adenoma, in all categories. The complications of hypercortisolism lead to a rise in mortality of patients with CS, being four times the one of the general population [65, 66].

The rise of mortality and the necessity to apply treatment to various complications and comorbidities of CS are additional factors for the reduction of QoL in CS [67-76].

Hypertension, coagulopathy, and metabolic syndrome are the main causes of cardiovascular risk, characterized by arterial rigidity and premature atherosclerosis. The cardiovascular risk increases along the seriousness and length of the hypercortisolism. Despite studies do not demonstrate the increase in the cardiovascular mortality after the cure; the morbidity remains because, besides the persistence of the risk factors, such as hypertension and the Metabolic Syndrome, the recovery of immunity after cure contributes to the atherogenesis [77-79].

Patients with DM have a progressive decline in QoL, aggravated by their complications and comorbidities. In fact, the highly prevalent cardiovascular complications and comorbidities (such as HAS and cardiac ischemic disease) in diabetic patients are the most important factors in the fall of the QoL in these patients [80].

Other complications of CS are bone diseases, especially osteoporosis, but also osteoarthritis and osteonecrosis due to the action of glucocorticoids in the bone formation and reabsorption, principally in the trabecular bone (spine). Despite that, after the cure and with the treatment with bisphosphonates, there is a recovery of the bone mass in those with osteoporosis (conversely, in osteoarthritis, there is no improvement after cure) [67-70, 79, 81-85].

The reduction in bone mass is related to the increase in the risk of fractures. The latter constitute an important cause of physical incapacity, with pain and mood alterations and result in an impairment of QoL [67, 68, 86].

Also, in CS there is a propensity to nephrolithiasis and kidney failure which improves with the remission of the disease [71, 72]. CS causes atrophy of certain cerebral areas, leading to mental disturbs, such as depression and cognitive decline, which generally are solved with the cure of CS (even with reversion of atrophy). Despite that, some damages are permanent [73-75, 87-95].

While patients with CS are immunosuppressed with a higher risk of infections, those who were cured have predisposition to self-immune diseases [96, 97].

The hypercortisolism suppresses the TSH and gonadotropins leading to hypothyroidism and hypogonadism (usually reversible with the cure, except when a pituitary gland lesion occurs) [4, 18, 79, 98]. The impairment of the QoL in hypothyroidism and hypogonadism is the object of other chapters present in this publication.

Other disorders common after the CD treatment are the hypocortisolism and the GH deficiency [99-101]. The reduction of QoL in patients with GH deficit is also object of discussion of another chapter in this publication.

The QoL of patients with CS is severely compromised due to the clinical complications during the permanence of the disease and after its remission [62].

Effects of Treatment on Quality of Life

As mentioned before, the treatment of Cushing's syndrome is conducted through surgery mostly but also with drug therapy and radiotherapy. Despite that, not all patients reach the remission of hypercortisolism. Sometimes, the cortisol levels are normalized without reaching the physiological pattern of the liberation cycle of it. However, in patients that present normalized cortisol levels or even hypocortisolism, other manifestations may occur. Therefore, despite usually demonstrating considerable clinical improvement, they will present complications reminiscent of hypercortisolism and/or developed after its remission [4, 18, 62, 79, 98]. After the remission of CS, the Metabolic Syndrome persists in a great number of patients, where the persistence of visceral obesity and insulin resistance seems fundamental [78, 102].

Van Aken et al. [103] developed a study in Holland to evaluate the quality of life of patients with CS treated by transsphenoidal surgery and, if necessary, by means of additional treatments. The 48 patients had a criteria of cure and were evaluated according to deficits of pituitary hormones: performance of pituitary-adrenal axis, GH, free T4, testosterone (in men), and estradiol (in women with premenopausal amenorrhea). In the case of some hormone deficiency, the patients received replacement therapy. This group was compared with control group patients of the same region and with patients of other European studies. In 52% of patients, hormone replacement therapy was conducted; 38% had multiple hormonal deficiencies. QoL of patients with CS history and of the control group was evaluated through questionnaires (SF-36, NHP, MFI-20 e HADS). The patients with history of CS demonstrated a QoL significantly inferior to the ones of the control group. Patients who needed radiotherapy did not present reduction in the QoL in relation to those who did not need it. Patients with hypopituitarism had worse QoL, but there was no difference between patients with only one deficiency and patients with multiple hormonal deficiencies. On the other hand, patients without hypopituitarism did not have a QoL significantly worse than the control population, except on the questions related to physical fatigue. Other independent determinant factors of QoL were age, age at diagnosis, and female gender.

Quality of Life in Children with Cushing's Syndrome

Besides the damages common to adults, the CS suppresses the linear growth in children [104]. Keil et al. (2009) [105] evaluated the QoL in 40 children with CS (34 with pituitary tumors, submitted to transsphenoidal surgery; and 6 with adrenal tumor, submitted to adrenalectomy) before and one year after the cure. HRQoL data were analyzed and 26 out of the 40 patients went through cognitive evaluation. Patients over 10 years old and parents of the patients below this age indicated before and after treatment which signs and symptoms (out of a list of 34) of CS were present. The children had height and bone mass index (BMI) determined. The possibility of association between the recovery of the hypothalamic-pituitary adrenal axis (HPA), the degree and/or length of hypercortisolism, and the BMI with HRQL scores was evaluated. Before treatment, the scores related to physical and psychosocial functions were significantly inferior to the North American population, presenting substantial improvement after treatment. Despite that, many patients remained significantly below the North American scores. There was no significant difference between pre- and post- treatment in relation to the behavior and emotional behavior scores, nor evidence of association between the QoL and the length of the CS, urinary cortisol levels or plasma free cortisol at midnight, which goes against the findings from other authors. Among the 40 patients, 26 completed the cognitive evaluation which evaluated the verbal, execution, and complete IQ. No deficit on the cognitive function was verified during the evaluation before the cure; nevertheless this function declined after the cure. Older patients experienced a smaller decline in the cognitive function - the older than 14 years subgroup had just a verbal function deficit, while the younger than 14 years old had a significantly drop in all the parameters. The incomplete HPA recovery after one year of treatment was related to the higher impairment of the general, emotional, and physical health in relation to the North American norms (gauged by sex). There were associations between the alterations on the scores of the physical functions after treatment (a year) and the BMI (ratifying the findings in obtained in studies on QoL in obese children) [106-108].

Before treatment, the most frequent symptoms related were weight gain, moon face, headaches, prominent abdomen, fatigue, alteration of humor, acne, buffalo hump, increased irritability, frustration, sensation of being fat and ugly, and anger. There was important improvement after treatment. Despite that, symptoms like headaches and fatigue remained [105].

Quality of Life in Pregnant Women with Cushing's Syndrome

By the 11th week of pregnancy, the cortisol levels start to rise [109] considering that, by the end of pregnancy and beginning of puerperium, there is a significant drop of the inhibition of the dexametasone over the levels of plasma free cortisol and urinary cortisol [110, 111]– the answer to cortisol and exogenous is diminished [112].

The occurrence of CS in pregnancy is rare and of difficult diagnosis. The CS inhibits the ovarian cycle and many of the manifestations of the CS are normal on gestation [113, 114]. Among pregnant women, adrenal CS is more common than CD; opposed to what is observed in the general population [3, 114-120].

The CS during pregnancy is related to various maternal complications, mostly to hypertension, diabetes and glucose intolerance, but also, in smaller proportion, bad cicatrization, osteoporosis, psychiatric disturbs, cardiac insufficiency, and death [114, 116, 121-125]. The fetal complications are: spontaneous abortion, prematurity (main accountant for the morbidity and mortality), intrauterine growth delay [116], respiratory insufficiency [126], intra-ventricular hemorrhage [127], HELLP syndrome (patients with serious preeclampsia that occurs with hemolysis, rise of hepatic enzymes and thrombocytopenia) [128] and, rarely, adrenal insufficiency and congenital malformations - despite that there are no signs of hypercortisolism (due to the degradation of this hormone by the placenta) [114, 126].

The complications are more important in the CS than in the CD [115, 117].

Conclusion

Although there are no specific questionnaires to the evaluation of QoL in patients with CS, it has been analyzed in many studies through unspecific questionnaires. These studies have shown that QoL is extensively impaired, even after treatment.

Treatment of CS, besides reducing mortality, is able to improve clinical conditions and QoL, but it remains reduced due to the complications of hypercortisolism and those developed after its remission.

References

[1] Girald F. P. Recent challenges in the diagnosis of Cushing's syndrome. *Horm Res.*, 2009, 71 (Suppl 1): 123-127.

[2] Pivonello R., De Martino M. C., De Leo M., et al. Cushing's syndrome. *Endocrinol Metab Clin North Am.*, 2008, 37:135-149.

[3] Newell-Price J., Trainer P., Besser G. M., Grossman A. The diagnosis and differential diagnosis of Cushing's syndrome and pseudo-Cushing's states. *Endocrine Rev.*, 1998, 19:647-672.

[4] Newell-Price J., Bertagna X., Grossman A. B., Nieman L. K. Cushing's syndrome. *Lancet*, 2006, 367:1605-1617.

[5] Vilar L., Freitas M. C., Faria M., et al. Pitfalls in the diagnosis of Cushing's syndrome. *Arq Brasil Endocrinol Metab.*, 2007, 51:1207-1216.

[6] Afandi B., Toumeh M. S., Saadi H. F. Cushing's syndrome caused by unsupervised use of ocular glucocorticoids. *Endocr Pract.*, 2003, 9:526-529.

[7] Gupta P., Goyal S., Gonzalez-Mendoza L. E., et al. Corticotropin-independent Cushing's syndrome in a child with na ovarian tumor misdiagnosed as nonclassic congenital adrenal hyperplasia. *Endocr Pract.*, 2008, 4:875-879.

[8] Jain S. H., Sadow P. M., Nosé V., Dluhy R. G. Medscape. A patient with ectopic cortisol production derived from malignant testicular masses. *Nat Clin Pract Endocrinol Metab.*, 2008, 4:695-700.

[9] Bourdeau I., Lampron A., Costa M. H., et al. Adrenocorticotropic hormone-independent Cushing's syndrome. *Curr Opin Endocrinol Diabetes Obes.*, 2007, 14:219-225.

[10] Costa M. H. S., Lacroix A. Cushing's syndrome secondary to ACTH-independent macronodular adrenal hyperplasia. *Arq Brasil Endocrinol Metab.*, 2007, 51: 1226-1237.

[11] Stewart P. M. The adrenal cortex. In: Kronenberg H. M., et al. (eds.) *Williams Textbook of Endocrinology.* 11th ed. Philadelphia, USA: W. B. Saunders; 2008:445-504.

[12] Becker M., Aron C. D. Ectopic ACTH syndrome and CRH-mediated Cushing's syndrome. *Endocrinol Metab Clin North Am.*, 1994, 23:585-606.

[13] Nieman L. K., Biller B. M., Findling J. W., et al. The diagnosis of Cushing's syndrome: an Endocrine Society Clinical Pratice Guideline. *J Clin Endocrinol Metab.*, 2008, 93:1525-1540.

[14] Magiaku M. A., Mastorakos G., Oldfield E. H., et al. Cushing's syndrome in children and adolescents. Presentation, diagnosis and therapy. *N Engl J Med.*, 1994, 31:629-637.

[15] Chan L. F., Storr H. L., Grossman A.B., Savage M. O. Pediatric Cushing's syndrome: Clinical features, diagnosis, and treatment. *Arq Brasil Endocrinol Metab.*, 2007, 51:1261-1271.

[16] Mansmann G., Lau J., Balk E., et al. The clinically unapparent adrenal mass: Update in diagnosis and management. *Endocr Rev.*, 2004 25, p. 309-40.

[17] Vilar L., Freitas M. C., Canadas V., et al. Adrenal incidentalomas diagnostic evaluation and long-term follow-up. *Endocr Pract.*, 2008, 14:269-78.

[18] Arnaldi G., Angeli A., Atkinson A. B., et al. Diagnosis and complications of Cushing's syndrome: a consensus statement. *J Clin Endocrinol Metab.*, 2003, 88:5593-5602.

[19] Albiger N. M. E., Scaroni C. M., Mantero F. Cyclic Cushing's syndrome: Na overview. *Arq Brasil Endocrinol Metab.*, 2007, 51:1253-1260.

[20] Miller J., Crapo L. The biochemical diagnosis of hypercortisolism. *Endocrinologist.*, 1994, 4:7-16.

[21] Terzolo M., Allasino B., Bosio S., et al. Hyperhomocysteinemia in patients with Cushing's syndrome. *J Clin Endocrinol Metab.*, 2004, 89:3743-3751.

[22] Castro M., Moreira A. C. Screening and diagnosis of Cushing's syndrome. *Arq Bras Endocrinol Metab.*, 2007, 51:1191-1198.

[23] Raff H. Salivary cortisol: an useful measurement in the diagnosis of Cushing's syndrome and the evaluation of hypothalamic-pituitary-adrenal axis. *Endocrinologist.* , 2000, 10:9-17.

[24] Bertagna X., Raux-Demay M. C., Guilhaume B., et al. Cushing's disease. In: Melmed S (ed). *The Pituitary***.** 2nd ed. Massachusetts, USA: Blackwell Science; 2002:496-560.

[25] Biller B. M., Grosman A. B., Stewart P. M., et al. Treatment of adrenocorticotropin-dependent Cushing's syndrome: a consensus statement. *J clin Endocrinol Metab.*, 2008, 93:2454-2462.

[26] Laws Jr E. R., Thapar K. Pituitary surgery. *Endocrinol Metab Clin North Am.* , 1999, 28:119-131.

[27] Vilar L., Naves L., Freitas M. C., et al. Tratamento medicamentoso dos tumores hipofisários. Parte II: Adenomas secretores de ACTH, TSH e

clinicamente não-funcionantes. *Arq Bras Endocrinol Metab.*, 2000, 44:455-470.

[28] Minnati G., Brada M. Radioherapy and radiosurgery for Cushing's disease. *Arq Bras Endocrinol Metab.*, 2007, 51:1373-1380.

[29] Young Jr W. F., Thompson G. B. Role for laparoscopic adrenalectomy in patients with Cushing's syndrome. *Arq Bras Endocrinol Metab.*, 2007, 51, p. 1349-1354.

[30] Wajchenberg B. L., Mendonça B. B., Liberman B., et al. Ectopic adrenocorticotropic hormone syndrome. *Endocr Rev.*, 1994, 15:752-787.

[31] Schell S. R., Camp E. R., Caridi J. G., Hawkins Jr I. F. Hepatic artery embolization for control of symptons, octreotide requirements, and tumor progression in metastatic tumors. *J Gastrointest Surg.*, 2002, 6:664-670.

[32] Sarmiento J. M., Heywood G., Rubin J., et al. Surgical Treatment of neuroendocrine metastases to the liver: a plea for resection to increase survival. *J Am Coll Surg.*, 2003, 197:29-37.

[33] Lehnert T. Liver transplantation for metastatic neuroendocrine carcinoma: an analysis of 130 patients. *Transplantation*, 1998, 66:1307-1312.

[34] Oberg K. Carcinoid tumors: molecular genetics, tumor biology, and update of diagnosis and treatment. *Curr Opin Oncol.*, 2002, 14:38-45.

[35] Della Torre S., Procopio G., Fusi A., et al. Current Treatments of neuroendocrine tumors role of biotherapy and chemotherapy. *Tumori*, 2033, 89: 111-116.

[36] Faiss S., Papa U. F., Bohmig M., et al. The International Lanreotide and Interferon Alfa Study Group. Prospective, randomized, multicenter trial on the antiproliferative effect of lanreotide, interferon alpha, and their combination for therapy of metastatic neuroendocrine gastroenteropancreatic tumors. *J Clin Oncol.*, 2003, 21:2689-2696.

[37] Bomanji J. B., Wong W., Gaze M. N., et al. Treatment of neuroendocrine tumours in adults with 131I-MIBG therapy. *Clin Oncol.*, 2003, 15:193-198.

[38] Trainer P. J., Besser M. Cushing`s syndrome: therapy directed at the adrenal glands. *Endocrinol Metab Clin North Am.*, 1994, 23:571-584.

[39] Klose M., Jorgensen K., Kristensen L. O. Characteristics of recovery of adrencortical function after treatment fo Cushing`s Syndrome due to pituitary or adrenal adenomas. *Clin Endocrinol.*, 2004, 61:394-399.

[40] Assalia A., Gagner M. Laparoscopic adrenalectomy. *Br J Surg*., 2004, 91:1259-1274.

[41] Gumbs A. A., Gagner M. Laparoscopic adrenalectomy. Best Pract. *Res Clin Endocrinol Metab*., 2006, 20:483-499.

[42] Rodríguez J. M., Parrilla P., Piñero A. Hipercortisolismos (síndrome de Cushing). En: Sitges-Serra A., Sancho J. J. (eds). *Cirugía endocrina. Guías clínicas de la asociación española de cirujanos*. Madrid, Spain: Aran Ediciones; 1997, 157-159.

[43] Czepielewski M. A., Rollin G. A. F. S. Carcinoma de Córtex Supra-renal. In: Coronho V, et al. (eds). *Tratado de endocrinologia e cirurgia endócrina*. Rio de Janeiro, Brazil: Guanabara Koogan; 2001:783-788.

[44] Pecori Giraldi F., Cavagnini F. Advances in the medical management of Cushing`s syndrome. *Exp Opin Pharmacother*., 2008, 9:2423-2433.

[45] Sonino N., Boscaro M., Fallo F. Pharmacologic management of Cushing syndrome: new targets for therapy. *Treat Endocrinol*., 2005, 4:87-94.

[46] Gómez R. M., Albiger N. E., Díaz A. G., Moncet D., Pitoia F., Bruno O. D. Effect of hypercortisolism control on high blood pressure in 71 patients with Cushing's syndrome. *Medicina (Buenos Aires)*, 2007, 67:439-444.

[47] Ware J. E., Sherbourne C. D. The MOS 36-item short-form health survey (SF-36). *Med Care*, 1992, 30:473–481.

[48] Ware J. E., Kosinski M. Interpreting SF-36 summary health measures: a response. *Qual Life Res.,* 2001, 10(5):405-413; discussion 415-420.

[49] Van der Zee K. I., Sanderman R., Heyink A. Comparison of two multidimensional measures of health status: the Nottingham Health Profile and the RAND 36-Item Health Survey 1.0. *Qual Life Res J*., 1996, 5:165–174.

[50] Hopman W. M., Verner J. Quality of life during and after inpatient stroke rehabilitation. *Stroke*, 2003, 34(3):801-805.

[51] Lai S. M., Perera S., Duncan P. W., Bode R. Physical and social functioning after stroke: comparison of the Stroke Impact Scale and Short Form-36. *Stroke*, 2003, 34(2):488-493.

[52] Anderson C., Laubsher S., Burns R. Validation of the short form 36 (SF-36) health survey questionnaire among stroke patients. *Stroke*, 1996, 27(10):1812-1816.

[53] Hunt S. M., McKenna S. P., McEwen J., Backett E. M., Williams J., Papp E. A quantitative approach to perceived health status: a validation study. *J Epidemiol Community Health*, 1980, 34(4):281–286.

[54] Hunt S. M., McEwen J. The development of a subjective health indicator. *Sociol Health Illn.*, 1980, 2:231–246.

[55] Hinz A., Klaiberg A., Schumacher J., Brahler E. The psychometric quality of the Nottingham Health Profile (NHP) in the general population. *Psychother Psychosom Med Psychol.*, 2003, 53:353–358.

[56] Teixeira-Salmela L. F., Magalhães L. C., Souza A. C., Lima M. C., Lima R. C. M., Goulart F. Adaptação do perfil de saúde de Nottingham: um instrumento simples de avaliação da qualidade de vida. *Cad Saúde Pública*, 2004, 20(4):905-914.

[57] Smets E. M., Garssen B., Bonke B., De Haes J. C. The Multidimensional Fatigue Inventory (MFI) psychometric qualities of an instrument to assess fatigue. *J Psychosom Res.*,1995, 39:315–325.

[58] Smets E. M., Visser M. R., Willems-Groot A. F., Garssen B., Schuster-Uitterhoeve A. L., De Haes J. C. Fatigue and radiotherapy: (B) experience in patients 9 months following treatment. *Br J Cancer*, 1998, 78:907–912.

[59] Zigmond A. S., Snaith R. P. The hospital anxiety and depression scale. *Acta Psychiatr Scand.*, 1983, 67:361–370.

[60] Sonino N., Fava G. A., Raffi A. R., Boscaro M., Fallo F. Clinical correlates of major depression in Cushing's disease. *Psychopathology*, 1990, 831:302–306.

[61] Kelly W. F. Psychiatric aspects of Cushing's syndrome. *Q J Med.*, 1996, 89:543–551.

[62] Pivonello R., De Martino M. C, De Leo M., Tauchmanovà L., Faggiano A., Lombardi G., Colao A. Cushing's syndrome: aftermath of the cure. *Arq Bras Endocrinol Metab.*, 2007, 51:1381-1391.

[63] Orth DN. Cushing's syndrome. *N Engl J Med.*, 1995, 332:791-803.

[64] Johnson M. D., Woodburn C. J., Vance M. L. Quality of Life in Patients with a Pituitary Adenoma. *Pituitary*, 2003, 6(2):81-87.

[65] Etxabe J., Vazquez J. A. Morbidity and mortality in Cushing's disease: an epidemiological approach. *Clin Endocrinol.*, 1994, 40:479-484.

[66] Lindholm J., Juul S., Jørgensen J. O., Astrup J., Bjerre P., Feldt-Rasmussen U., et al. Incidence and late prognosis of Cushing's syndrome: a population-based study. *J Clin Endocrinol Metab.*, 2001, 86:117-1123.

[67] Di Somma C., Pivonello R., Loche S., Faggiano A., Marzullo P., Di Sarno A., et al. Severe impairment of bone mass and turnover in Cushing's disease: comparison between childhood-onset and adulthood-onset disease. *Clin Endocrinol.*, 2002, 56:153-158.

[68] Tauchmanovà L., Pivonello R., Di Somma C., Rossi R., De Martino M. C., Camera L., et al. Bone demineralization and vertebral fractures in endogenous cortisol excess: role of disease etiology and gonadal status. *J Clin Endocrinol Metab.*, 2006, 91:1779-1784.

[69] Faggiano A., Pivonello R., Filippella M., Di Somma C., Orio Jr F., Lombard G., et al. Spine abnormalities and damage in patients cured from Cushing's disease. *Pituitary*, 2001, 4:153-161.

[70] Phillips K. A., Nance Jr E. P., Rodriguez R. M., Kaye J. J. Avascular necrosis of bone: a manifestation of Cushing's disease. *South Med J.*, 1986, 79:825-829.

[71] Faggiano A., Pivonello R., Melis D., Filippella M., Di Somma C., Peretta M., et al. Nephrolithiasis in Cushing's disease: prevalence, etiopathogenesis, and modification after disease cure. *J Clin Endocrinol Metab.* 2003, 88:2076-2080.

[72] Faggiano A., Pivonello R., Melis D., Alfieri R., Filippella M., Spagnuolo G., et al. Evaluation of circulating levels and renal clearance of natural amino acids in patients with Cushing's disease. *J Endocrinol Invest.*, 2002, 25:142-151.

[73] Sonino N., Fava G. A. Psychiatric disorders associated with Cushing's syndrome. Epidemiology, pathophysiology and treatment. *CNS Drugs,* 2001, 15:361-373.

[74] Bourdeau I., Bard C., Forget H., Boulanger Y., Cohen H., Lacroix A. Cognitive function and cerebral assessment in patients who have Cushing's syndrome. *Endocrinol Metab Clin North Am.*, 2005, 34:357-369.

[75] Mauri M., Sinforiani E., Bono G., Vignati F., Berselli M. E., Attanasio R., et al. Memory impairment in Cushing's disease. *Acta Neurol Scand.*, 1993, 87:52-5.

[76] Bourdeau I., Bard C., Noël B., Leclerc I., Cordeau M. P., Bélair M., et al. Loss of brain volume in endogenous Cushing's syndrome and its reversibility after correction of hypercortisolism. *J Clin Endocrinol Metab.*, 2002, 87:1949-1954.

[77] Pivonello R., Faggiano A., Lombardi G., Colao A. The metabolic syndrome and cardiovascular risk in Cushing's syndrome. *Endocrinol Metab Clin North Am.*, 2005, 34:327-329.

[78] Colao A., Pivonello R., Spiezia S., Faggiano A., Ferone D., Filippella M., et al. Persistence of increased cardiovascular risk in patients with Cushing's disease after five years of successful cure. *J Clin Endocrinol Metab.*, 1999, 84:2664-2672.

[79] Pivonello R., De Martino M. C., De Leo M., Lombardi G., Colao A. Cushing's syndrome. *Endocrinol Metab Clin North Am.*, 2008, 37(1):135-49.

[80] Costa Jr. A. C. M., Miranda M. P., Moura J. C., Martins C. F., Oliveira P. O., Cerqueira E. F. S., et al. Diabetes and Quality of life in Hospitalized Patients. *Endocr Rev.*, 2011, 32 (03_MeetingAbstracts):P1-526.

[81] Manning P. J., Evans M. C., Reid I. R. Normal bone mineral density following cure of Cushing's syndrome. *Clin Endocrinol.*, 1992, 36:229-234.

[82] Hermus A. R., Smals A. G., Swinkels L. M., Huysmans D. A., Pieters G. F., Sweep C. F., et al. Bone mineral density and bone turnover before and after surgical cure of Cushing's syndrome. *J Clin Endocrinol Metab.*, 1995, 80:2859-2865.

[83] Di Somma C., Pivonello R., Loche S., Faggiano A., Klain M., Salvatore M., et al. Effect of 2 years of cortisol normalization on the impaired bone mass and turnover in adolescent and adult patients with Cushing's disease: a prospective study. *Clin Endocrinol.*, 2003, 58:302-308.

[84] Kristo C., Jemtland R., Ueland T., Godang K., Bollerslev J. Restoration of the coupling process and normalization of bone mass following successful treatment of endogenous Cushing's syndrome: a prospective, long-term study. *Eur J Endocrinol.*, 2006, 154:109-118.

[85] Di Somma C., Colao A., Pivonello R., Klain M., Faggiano A., Tripodi F. S., et al. Effectiveness of chronic treatment with alendronate in the osteoporosis of Cushing's disease. *Clin Endocrinol.*, 1998, 48:655-662.

[86] Nascimento O. R., Cemin F. S., Morais M., Barroco R. S., Fujiki E. M., Milani C. Avaliação da qualidade de vida em pacientes com fratura da tíbia. *Acta Ortop Bra.*, 2009, 17(4):211-214.

[87] Momose K. J., Kjellberg R. N., Kliman B. High incidence of cortical atrophy of the cerebral and cerebellar hemispheres in Cushing's disease. *Radiology*, 1971, 99:341-348.

[88] Starkman M. N., Gebarski S. S., Berent S., Schteingart D. E. Hippocampal formation volume, memory dysfunction, and cortisol levels in patients with Cushing's syndrome. *Biol Psychiatry*, 1992, 32:756-765.

[89] Simmons N. E., Do H. M., Lipper M. H., Laws Jr E. R. Cerebral atrophy in Cushing's disease. *Surg Neurol.*, 2000, 53:72-6.

[90] Heinz E. R., Martinez J., Haenggeli A. Reversibility of cerebral atrophy in anorexia nervosa and Cushing's syndrome. *J Comput Assist Tomogr.*, 1977, 1:415-418.

[91] Starkman M. N., Giordani B., Gebarski S. S., Berent S., Schork M. A., Schteingart D. E. Decrease in cortisol reverses human hippocampal atrophy following treatment of Cushing's disease. *Biol Psychiatry*, 1999, 46:1595-1602.

[92] Starkman M. N., Schteingart D. E., Schork M. A. Cushing's syndrome after treatment: changes in cortisol and ACTH levels, and amelioration of the depressive syndrome. *Psychiatry Res.*, 1986, 19:177-188.

[93] Kelly W. F., Kelly M. J., Faragher B. A prospective study of psychiatric and psychological aspects of Cushing's syndrome. *Clin Endocrinol.*, 1996, 45:715-720.

[94] Dorn L. D., Burgess E. S., Friedman T. C., Dubbert B., Gold P. W., Chrousos G. P. The longitudinal course of psychopathology in Cushing's syndrome after correction of hypercortisolism. *J Clin Endocrinol Metab.*, 1997, 82:912-919.

[95] Merke D. P., Giedd J. N., Keil M. F., Mehlinger S. L., Wiggs E. A., Holzer S., et al. Children experience cognitive decline despite reversal of brain atrophy one year after resolution of Cushing's syndrome. J Clin Endocrinol Metab., 2005, 90:2531-2536.

[96] Dougherty T. F. Effect of hormones on lymphatic tissue. *Physiol Rev.* 1995, 232:379-401.

[97] Bateman A., Singh A., Kral T., Solomon S. The immune hypothalamic-pituitary-adrenal axis. *Endocr Rev.*, 1989, 10:92-112.

[98] Orth D. N. Cushing's syndrome. *N Engl J Med.* 1995, 332:791-803.

[99] Hughes N. R., Lissett C. A., Shalet S. M. Growth hormone status following treatment for Cushing's syndrome. *Clin Endocrinol.*, 1999, 51:61-66.

[100] Tzanela M., Karavitaki N., Stylianidou C., Tsagarakis S., Thalassinos N.C. Assessment of GH reserve before and after successful treatment of adult patients with Cushing's syndrome. *Clin Endocrinol.*, 2004, 60:309-314, 2004.

[101] Pecori Giraldi F., Andrioli M., De Marinis L., Bianchi A., Giampietro A., De Martin M., et al. Significant GH deficiency after long-term cure by surgery in adult patients with Cushing's disease. *Eur J Endocrinol.*, 2007, 156:233-239.

[102] Faggiano A., Pivonello R., Spiezia S., De Martino M. C., Filippella M., Di Somma C., et al. Cardiovascular risk factors and common carotid

artery caliber and stiffness in patients with Cushing's disease during active disease and 1 year after disease remission. *J Clin Endocrinol Metab.*, 2003, 88:2527-2533.

[103] Van Aken M. O., Pereira A. M., Biermasz N. R., van Thiel S. W., Hoftijzer H. C., Smit J. W., et al. Quality of life in patients after long-term biochemical cure of Cushing's disease. *J Clin Endocrinol Metab.*, 2005, 90(6):3279-3286.

[104] Batista D. L., Riar J., Keil M., Stratakis C. A. Diagnostic tests for children who are referred for the investigation of Cushing syndrome. *Pediatrics,* 2007, 120:e575–e586.

[105] Keil M. F., Merke D. P., Gandhi R., Wiggs E. A., Obunse K., Stratakis C. A.. Quality of life in children and adolescents 1-year after cure of Cushing syndrome: a prospective study. *Clin Endocrinol.*, 2009, 71(3):326-333.

[106] Swallen K. C., Reither E. N., Haas S. A., et al. Overweight, obesity, and health related quality of life among adolescents: the National Longitudinal Study of Adolescent Health. *Pediatrics*, 2005, 115:340–347.

[107] Modi A. C., Loux T. J., Bell S. K., et al. Weight-specific health-related quality of life in adolescents with extreme obesity. *Obesity,* 2008, 16:2266-2271.

[108] Fallon E. M., Tanofsky-Kraff M., Norman A. C., et al. Health-related quality of life in overweight and nonoverweight black and white adolescents. *J Pediatrics*, 2005, 147:443–450.

[109] Demey-Ponsart E., Foidart J. M., Sulon J., Sodoyez J. C. Serum CBG, free and total cortisol and circadian patterns of adrenal function in normal pregnancy. *J Steroid Biochem.*, 1982, 16:165-169.

[110] Sheeler L. R. Cushing's syndrome and pregnancy. *Endocrinol Metab Clin North Am.,* 1994, 23:619-627.

[111] Wallace C., Toth E. L., Lewanczuk R. Z., Siminoski K. Pregnancy-induced Cushing's syndrome in multiple pregnancies. *J Clin Endocrinol Metab.*, 1996, 81:15-21.

[112] Schulte H. M., Weisner D., Allolio B. The corticotrophin releasing hormone test in late pregnancy: lack of adrenocorticotrophin and cortisol response. *Clin Endocrinol.*, 1990, 33:99-106.

[113] Sheeler L. R. Cushing's syndrome and pregnancy. *Endocrinol Metab Clin North Am.*, 1994, 23:619-27.

[114] Lindsay J. R., Nieman L. K. The hypothalamic-pituitary-adrenal axis in pregnancy: Challenges in disease detection and treatment. *Endocr Rev.* 2005, 26:775-799.

[115] Aron D. C., Schnall A. M., Sheeler L. R. Cushing's syndrome and pregnancy. *Am J Obstet Gynecol.*, 1990, 162:244-252.

[116] Buescher M. A., McClamrock H. D., Adashi E. Y. Cushing's syndrome in pregnancy. *Obstet Gynecol.*, 1992, 79:130-137.

[117] Pickard J., Jochen A. L., Sadur C. N., Hofeldt F. D. Cushing's syndrome in pregnancy. *Obstet Gynecol Surv.*, 1990, 45:87-93.

[118] Invitti C., Giraldi F. P., de Martin M., Cavagnini F. Diagnosis and management of Cushing's syndrome: results of an Italian multicentre study. Study group of the Italian Society of Endocrinology on the pathophysiology of the hypothalamic-Pituitary-Adrenal Axis. *J Clin Endocrinol Metab.,* 1999, 84(2):440-448.

[119] Vilar L., Naves L. A., Freitas M. C., Moura E., Canadas V., Leal E., et al. Endogenous Cushing's syndrome: Clinical and laboratorial features in 73 cases. *Arq Bras Endocrinol Metab.*, 2007, 51:566-574.

[120] Casson I. F., Davis J. C., Jeffreys R. V., Silas J. H., Williams J., Belchetz P. E. Successful management of Cushing's disease during pregnancy by transsphenoidal adenectomy. *Clin Endocrinol.*, 1987, 27:423-428.

[121] Finkenstedt G., Gasser R. W., Hofle G., Lhotta K., Kolle D., Gschwendtner A., et al. Pheochromocytoma and sub-clinical Cushing's syndrome during pregnancy: Diagnosis, medical pre-treatment and cure by laparoscopic unilateral adrenalectomy. *J Endocrinol Invest.*, 1999, 22:551-557.

[122] Mellor A., Harvey R. D., Pobereskin L. H., Sneyd J. R. Cushing's disease treated by trans-sphenoidal selective adenomectomy in mid-pregnancy. *Br J Anaesth.*, 1998, 80:850-852.

[123] Tajika T., Shinozaki T., Watanabe H., Yangawa T., Takagishi K. Case report of a Cushing's syndrome patient with multiple pathologic fractures during pregnancy. *J Orthop Sci.*, 2002, 7:498-500.

[124] Kamiya Y., Okada M., Yoneyama A., Jin-no Y., Hibino T., Watanabe O., et al. Surgical successful treatment of Cushing's syndrome in a pregnant patient complicated with severe cardiac involvement. *Endocr J.*, 1988, 45:499-504.

[125] Bevan J. S., Gough M. H., Gillmer M. D., Burke C. W. Cushing's syndrome in pregnancy: the timing of definitive treatment. *Clin Endocrinol.,* 1987, 27:225-233.

[126] Cabezon C., Bruno O. D., Cohen M., Garcia S., Gutman R.A. Twin pregnancy in a patient with Cushing's disease. *Fertil Steril.*, 1999, 72:371-372.

[127] Castro M., Elias P. C., Quidute A. R., Halah F. P., Moreira A. C. Out-patient screening for Cushing's syndrome: The sensitivity of the combination of circadian rhythm and overnight dexamethasone suppression salivary cortisol tests. *J Clin Endocrinol Metab.*, 1999, 84:878-882.

[128] Viardot A., Huber P., Puder J. J., Zulewski H., Keller U., Muller B. Reproducibility of nighttime salivary cortisol and its use in the diagnosis of hypercortisolism compared with urinary free cortisol and overnight dexamethasone suppression test. *J Clin Endocrinol Metab.*, 2005, 90:5730-5736.

In: Quality of Life in Endocrine Diseases ISBN: 978-1-63463-911-8
Editor: Erika Cesar de Oliveira Naliato © 2015 Nova Science Publishers, Inc.

Chapter 6

Hypogonadism and Quality of Life

Michael P. Miranda and Erika C. O. Naliato*
Center of Studies Ricardo A T Castilho of the Teresópolis Medical Association, Brazil

Abbreviations

A-RHDQoL	Age Related Hormone Deficiency-Dependent Quality of Life Questionnaire
BMD	Bone Mineral Density
BMI	Body mass index
FSH	Follicle-stimulating hormone
LH	Luteinizing hormone
MRS	Menopause Rating Scale
MENQOL	Menopause Specific Quality of Life Questionnaire
PSA	Prostate-specific antigen
QoL	Quality of Life
SF-36	Medical Outcome Study Short Form 36

* Correspondence to: erikanaliato@uol.com.br.

Introduction

Hypogonadism is characterized by the reduction in the production of sexual hormones by the gonads. It may be classified as primary and secondary. [1]

Primary hypogonadism is also called hypogonadotropic hypogonadism. This kind of hypogonadism is characterized by the association of low levels of gonadal hormones with high levels of the follicle-stimulating hormone (FSH) and luteinizing hormone (LH), demonstrating that the defects in the production of sexual hormones have gonadal origin despite adequate and even increased stimulus of the gonadotrophins [1]. Primary hypogonadism may arise from a chromosomal alteration, as in the Klinefelter and Turner Syndromes, or be acquired, as in the cases of viral orchitis, trauma, chemotherapy, or even derived from the natural ageing process characterized by the menopause. All these possible causes make primary hypogonadism a very common condition in medical practice [1, 2]. In men, it is proven that advanced age, Diabetes Mellitus type II, and obesity may predispose to hypogonadism. Data from the year 2006 suggest that four million North American men suffer of hypogonadism [3]. The authors suggested a tendency to an elevation of this number due to the ageing of population and the increase in the incidence of Diabetes and obesity, which may cause the reduction of levels of plasma androgens [3].

In secondary hypogonadism, low levels of FSH and LH are found as a result of pituitary or hypothalamic alterations. The main causes are: (1) congenital, such as Kallman Syndrome and (2) acquired, such as hyperprolactinemia, Sheehan Syndrome, pituitary tumors, and disruption of the hypothalamic-pituitary axis resulting from radiotherapy or surgical treatment of a brain tumor [1,2].

When hypogonadism affects the patient during puberty, it prevents the normal development of the secondary sexual characters (pubarche, thelarche, and external genitalia growth), possibly presenting different patterns according to the etiology [4]. Women with hypogonadism in puberty may present primary amenorrhea [4, 5]. Adults with hypogonadism may have extremely varied clinical signals and symptomatology, including skin and mucosa alterations, hot flushes, osteopenia, and reduction of libido [4].

Men with androgenic deficiency may present complaints such as lack of energy and motivation in addition to sexual impotence and reduction of body hair [4]. Hypogonadal men also present increased cardiovascular risk independently of factors such as age, composition, and metabolic alterations [6, 7].

In women in perimenopause, the emotional symptoms present great importance, being very frequent the presence of anxiety, irritability, depression, reduction of libido in addition to difficulty of concentration, and decrease of memory and general well-being [8]. As observed in the masculine gender, in women, the hypogonadism has also been associated to the increase of cardiovascular risk [9, 10].

For the diagnosis, besides anamnesis and detailed physical exam, LH, FSH, testosterone and estradiol laboratory tests are also important. The presence of low levels of testosterone or estradiol and high levels of LH and FSH characterizes the primary hypogonadism [5]. If, besides the low levels of testosterone and estradiol, LH and FSH also present low or normal levels, the hypogonadism is secondary [5]. It is also necessary to check the levels of serum prolactin in order to exclude the hyperprolactinemia as the cause of secondary hypogonadism [5, 11].

The execution of a magnetic resonance specially focused of the sellar region is important for the visualization of possible lesions and presence of tumors [12]. The anatomic analysis of the genital tract must be done through pelvic echography or even laparoscopy [5]. Although not much used at the moment, another method described in the literature for the evaluation of patients of the feminine gender is the conjugated estrogens test (dose = 1.25 mg/day for 21 days), associated to medroxyprogesterone acetate (dose = 10 mg/day over the last 10 days). The negative result, in other words, the absence of bleeding, suggests the presence of an anatomical defect of the genital tract [5]. It is important to notice that this test is only indicated when the evaluation of hormonal levels is unavailable. The karyotype analysis may be requested for both genders, especially when hypogonadism is diagnosed during the development of the secondary sexual characteristics [2].

The treatment of hypogonadism in young people at the time of the development of the secondary sexual characteristics is done with replacement of gonadal hormones and must be initiated at the chronological age when this development usually occurs to avoid psychosocial disturbance on patients, such as low self-esteem and depression [13]. In boys, around the 13 years of age, the replacement with some kind of long duration testosterone must be initiated, such as testosterone enanthate on a dose of 50 to 100 mg intramuscular every 4 weeks, for an average period of 9 months; after which the dose must be increased to 200 to 300 mg every two or three weeks for the next years. In girls, the beginning of the therapy must be a little more precocious, around the 12 years of age, being made with ethynylestradiol 5 μg/day in oral administration and continuous for the first six months. After this period, the administration becomes cyclical over the first 21 days of each month, being increased to 10 μg/day. In this second phase, the progesterone is added to the estradiol on days 12 and 21 of the cycle, being the progesterone acetate the most-used formulation [13]. In post menopausal women, hormonal replacement can be made with estrogen and progesterone [14, 15]. There are controversies in relation to the use of androgens in post menopausal women, as some authors consider it beneficial for the treatment of the reduced libido and other symptoms, but there is no completely clear definition about its indications [14, 15].

All patients submitted to hormonal replacement must be carefully followed-up [16, 17, 18]. Many studies discuss the risks of androgenic replacement for the appearance of prostate cancer [19]. Despite that, due to the different conclusions presented by these studies, no relation has been established. However, before beginning the replacement, there must be an investigation with PSA tests, digital rectal examination, and even prostate biopsy as hormonal replacement may accelerate the development of a pre-existent carcinoma [19]. Continual monitoring is indicated for patients under hormonal replacement treatment [19]. In women, estrogenic replacement also presents risks [16, 17]. High profile studies suggest a proportional rise of the risk of developing breast cancer when the hormonal replacement surpasses five years, presenting a maximum increase of this risk after the 15 years of hormonal therapy [20]. Another risk of the estrogenic replacement, already known for more than 20 years, is the endometrium cancer [21]. Despite that, this risk may be minimized or even abolished if the administration of a progesterone is added to the estrogenic therapy for, at least, 10 days in the month or even in continual use. Therapies with the addition of progesterone for less than 10 days present some reduction of this risk but are much less effective [21].

Quality of Life in Women with Hypogonadism - Menacme

Quality of life (QoL) was defined by the World Health Organization as the individual's perception of their position in life, in the context of culture and system of values in which they live and in relation to their objectives, expectations, standards and preoccupations [22].

In young women with hypogonadism, the majority of the works available in the literature study the QoL of patients with Turner Syndrome. No specific questionnaire for the evaluation of the QoL in these patients was found and, despite SF-36 questionnaire (*Medical Outcome Study Short Form 36*) being one of the most used, there is no standardization in the studies, with many using their own questionnaires.

Low stature, despite being cited by the majority of the works, was not considered one of the most important determining factors of the QoL by the majority of the patients with Turner Syndrome, not even implying in a reduction of the QoL scores in some studies [23, 24, 25]. Despite that, the treatment for patients to reach higher stature continues to be indicated because the absence of treatment with the growth hormone or oxandrolone implied in more reference of sleep-related problems and social isolation by part of the patients [24]. Nevertheless, in a Japanese study, a significant amount of patients complained about the difficulty in finding clothes and shoes that match their stature [26]. The otologic disturbs, present in a good part of patients, surprisingly, were pointed out as the main causes of loss of QoL, having to be closely managed by specialists [23, 27].

Another great difficulty mentioned by patients was infertility. A great amount of them related feeling devastated at the moment when they received the news about their infertility, being a sensitive topic even after their better assimilation of the information [25]. The diagnosis of infertility is pointed as a modifier on the manner these women relate to men, as they fear the rejection when communicating their impossibility of bearing children [25]. The infertility condition must be followed by a multiprofessional team in order to reduce its impact on the lives of these women, because their relationship with men, the development of sexuality, the age when they start to have dates, and their first sexual relation are important in the determination of the QoL and their self-esteem [25, 27]. Patients who had puberty induced after their 15 years of age present significantly lower general health perception scores [23].

Another important finding that deserves the attention of the specialists is the growing number of patients with disorders on the sexual development who refer to damaged QoL, mental suffering, and suicidal thoughts when patients with Turner Syndrome are compared to control groups [28].

Hypogonadism in Men before and during Development of Secondary Sexual Characters

The presence of hypogonadism in young men during the period of development of secondary sexual characteristics may have negative influence in many aspects. Despite that, few studies have been conducted aiming at evaluating the most common alterations. The majority deals with patients with Klinefelter Syndrome.

As it is observed concerning the Turner Syndrome, there are no specific questionnaires for the evaluation of the QoL of these patients. Therefore, each study uses one or various questionnaires, which makes the identification of a pattern of alteration of QoL difficult or even the definition of a more prevalent questionnaire.

In the Klinefelter Syndrome, the patients present an XXY karyotype. In a study that evaluated the QoL of these patients in testosterone replacement therapy, it was found a more pronounced reduction of the QoL in the physical, social, and psychological subscales in addition to the reduction in seven out of the eight subscales evaluated on the SF-36 questionnaire (*36-Item Short Form Health Survey*) [29]. Nevertheless, the differences in the scales of QoL in the masculine population taken as reference for the study and the patients with Klinefelter decrease when the educational level is higher, even being similar when the patients present a Bachelor's or Master's degree [29].

Other studies also found alterations in the social interactions of people with Klinefelter. These patients experience more difficulty to relate themselves with others, especially during childhood. Many boys present shyness, being very introspective, avoiding more energetic children‘s play and crying easily when being the victim of more aggressive playing or bullying [30].

An important disorder in the development of patients with Klinefelter refers to the development of linguistic abilities, which may have a negative influence on their social relationships. These patients demonstrate depressed verbal ability, with a higher difficulty when the use of auditory memory, language comprehension and expressive ability are necessary [31]. Data demonstrate that up to 65% of patients with Klinefelter present language difficulties [32], with the necessity of specific therapy in more than half of the patients [30]. Other important disorders found in patients with Klinefelter, with a higher prevalence than in the general population, are disorders of attention deficit and hyperactivity and of the autistic spectrum [32]. An evaluation by the pediatric psychiatrist is advised, preferably before the 10 years of age in all patients with Klinefelter to obtain the precocious diagnosis and prevent that the necessary treatments start late. Besides that, the early diagnosis may protect these children from possible adverse environmental influences [32].

In a study developed to determine the most common sexual problems in patients with Klinefelter, it can be concluded that, between all the complaints, the only one which presented significantly increased prevalence in these patients was the hypoactive sexual drive [33]. The possible cause may be the hypogonadism itself and not specifically the Klinefelter Syndrome. The first-choice treatment for this alteration is the testosterone replacement [33].

The physical alterations presented by the patients with hypogonadism represent an important influence in the QoL. Patients affected by gynecomastia are socially more anxious and have a reduction in QoL. The absence of body and/or facial hair is related to higher levels of social anxiety. In addition, patients with micropenis, a relatively common finding in the Klinefelter Syndrome, present significantly lower results of self-esteem and QoL, added to higher social anxiety and depression [34].

Due to all these possible alterations, the proper follow-up of the patients with hypogonadism is important, with hormonal replacement in the adequate moment, aiming at reducing the physical effect of the condition, added to psychiatric treatment with pediatric specialist in order to treat the disorders and promote higher self-acceptance by the patients. Besides, it is necessary to supply specialized help to overcome the problems in learning and language domain.

Hypogonadism in Elderly Women

The main group of patients representing women who present hypogonadism after the development of the secondary sexual characteristics is that formed by women who reach menopause. A specific questionnaire was created to evaluate the symptoms of the menopause, the MRS, *Menopause Rating Scale*. Besides, there is a questionnaire developed for the evaluation of the QoL in these patients. The MENQOL, *Menopause Specific Quality of Life Questionnaire*, is a self-administrable questionnaire, developed by the Department of Family and Community Medicine of the University of Toronto, in Canada [35].

Every woman who lives long enough will present menopause and the symptoms presented by these women are very diverse. There are even differences in the symptomatology of the menopause when different ethnical groups are compared [36, 37]. The main symptoms related by women are presented in the table below:

Table 1. Main symptoms related by women in peri and post menopause

Vaginal dryness	Depressive humor
Muscular and joints discomfort	Sexual problems
Physical and mental exhaustion	Heart discomfort
Sleeping problems	Urinary problems
Hot flushes and sweat	Headaches
Irritability	Fatigue
Anxiety	

Table adapted from Rahman et al. 2011 [36].

Although these symptoms are always present, independently of the population in question, their incidence and severity differ according to the studied population. In studies carried in Asian countries, such as Bangladesh and Nepal, the most common symptoms were fatigue, headaches, muscular and joint discomfort, physical and mental exhaustion, and sleeping problems. Conversely, studies developed in Western countries reveal a higher incidence of hot flashes and night sweats [36, 38]. It is not probable that these alterations are secondary to the differences in the habits of life of each population because in an extensive study developed in the United States comparing Caucasian, African American, Hispanic, and Asian women, important ethnic differences were also found. This study showed that between Caucasian, African American, and Hispanic women, temperature alterations constituted the main symptom, while the majority of the Asian women mentioned reduced libido. The hot flashes were one of the symptoms mostly mentioned by Caucasian, African American, and Hispanic women, while, between the Asian women, the same did not figure even in the ten most frequent symptoms. Urinary nocturnal problems reached more Caucasian and African American women, while muscular and joint discomfort were more common in Caucasian and Asian women. The reduction of sexual interest was mentioned only by Hispanic and Asian women and weight gain was not an important complaint among Caucasian women only [37].

Another important discussion concerns the severity of the symptoms. Between all the symptoms, the hot flashes were the one classified by women as severe or very severe. Other symptoms also considered severe were depression, vaginal dryness, anxiety, and irritability [38]. Between ethnicities, the Hispanic women presented a higher amount of total symptoms, physical, psychological, and psychosomatic, while the Asian women referred the lowest amount of symptoms between the ethnicities. In addition, Hispanic women presented the highest severity of the symptoms followed by Caucasian, African-American and, finally, Asian women [37].

One of the main symptoms mentioned by women, the hot flashes or heat waves, has great negative influence in the QoL of patients with menopause. Besides the discomfort it causes during the days, it is also related with the decrease in the sleep quality of these women. An 80% index of insomnia was found between women who mentioned having severe hot flashes. It is also suggested that hot flashes should be researched in women with insomnia as many of them present an improvement in sleep quality with the treatment [39]. One valid solution to the treatment of hot flashes is weight loss. Women who obtained weight loss, BMI and abdominal circumference reductions presented an improvement of the discomfort caused by hot flashes [40]. And, despite many studies associating a higher BMI with a higher incidence of hot flashes, this mechanism is not yet comprehended, as it is known that women with higher concentration of adipose tissue present higher concentration of estrogens due to the aromatization that occurs on adipocytes [40].

Other sleep alterations not related to hot flushes were also found in women in the menopause, influencing negatively the QoL of these patients. Significant improvement in disturbs related to sleep fragmentation were found in women who started hormonal replacement. However, the mechanisms of this association have not been defined yet [41].

The urogenital alterations have great importance in the QoL of the patients in peri- and post menopause because, besides their physical implications, many times their psychological impact is rather strong in these women. Between the urogenital symptoms, the most common are vaginal dryness, pain or discomfort during the sexual act, and vaginal itchiness [42, 43]. Patients of every ethnicity refer that these symptoms influence their sexual life causing reduction of libido, making vaginal sex a painful experience, and causing these patients to avoid entering into a new relationship due to the fear of pain during the sexual act [42]. Complaints about pain during the sexual act are more common in diabetic women with low BMI and higher vaginal pH [43]. Vaginal dryness is more prevalent in non- Caucasian women, with lower BMI, sexually active, diabetic, and vaginal colonization by enterococci [43]. Other problems encountered in the everyday lives of these women are related to irritation, which prevent them from remaining seated for a long time, and even stay in public places over extensive periods of time due to the necessity of a private environment to soften the itching [42]. The lack of knowledge about the urogenital symptoms of the menopause in addition to the idea that these symptoms are a signal of ageing and body deterioration are responsible for causing feeling of depression and frustration in these women [42]. Despite the relevance of these symptoms, half of the women present an improvement in them without hormonal replacement therapy [43]. An important information to the health professionals is that many women revealed being reluctant in discussing these symptoms, even with the health professionals [42]. Considering this, it is necessary to direct the anamnesis of these patients in order to reveal the presence of these alterations.

Health professionals must stimulate women with menopause symptoms to practice physical exercises regularly. In women who practice exercises, improvement in the QoL and in the psychological aspects secondary to the reduction of the symptoms of the menopause occur [44]. When aerobic exercises were compared to resistance ones, both resulted in an improvement of the QoL, psychological health, and menopause symptoms, with some advantage of the aerobic exercises [44].

Another aspect that must be amply approached by health professionals is the educational intervention on patients with menopause. Women who received education about menopause and its symptomatology obtained significant improvement in the QoL, with reduction of menopause problems and their intensity [45].

The menopause is one of the most important causes for the reduction of the QoL in women and, as a result, must be approached in an integral manner by the health professionals. Only by this means the patients will manage to go through this phase more calmly, facing it as part of the natural ageing process and not as a disease, reducing the deleterious effects over the physical and mental health of these women.

Hypogonadism in Men after the Secondary Sexual Development

This group is represented especially by elderly men who, with the reduction of the testosterone plasma levels related to age progression, reach the andropause. Other patients also included within this group but with fewer works analyzing their QoL are men who experience a reduction in the levels of testosterone while still young or middle-aged, being patients treated for cancer an example of this group.

Multiple studies point to an important reduction in the QoL in elderly men with hypogonadism.

There is a specific questionnaire for the evaluation of the QoL in these patients known as *Age-Related Hormone Deficiency-Dependent Quality of Life Questionnaire* (A-RHDQoL). This questionnaire analyses many aspects, among them: family, social, work, sexual life, physical abilities, appearance, vigor, sleep, pain, psychological aspects, such as trust and motivation, in addition to health, fertility, concentration, and capacity of doing domestic activities. By the end, there is an area for free commentaries where it is asked about any other form in which hormonal deficiency due to age that may reduce the QoL. Despite that, its application is still very restricted. In addition to A-RHDQoL, other questionnaires and physical tests are used, intending to analyze the multiple health areas of the men affected by hypogonadism. The SF-36 questionnaire (*Short-Form Health Survey*) is applied by the main studies involving elderly hypogonadic men [46].

An important alteration found on the hypogonadism is the anemia secondary to the reduction of free testosterone. Conversely, patients treated with hormonal replacement evolve with the increase of hemoglobin and hematocrits levels [47, 48, 49, 50]. In a study developed by Thein et al. (2009) in elderly men with anemia, it was demonstrated a reduction of various domains of the SF-36 questionnaire [51]. Despite that, this relation has not yet been demonstrated in the anemia secondary to hypogonadism and may not be too relevant in patients without other associated comorbidities, because, as demonstrated by Ly et al. (2001), the red series levels are almost always under the limits of normality, even before the beginning of the hormonal replacement treatment [49].

Another important finding indicated by multiple works, is the reduction in the Bone Mineral Density (BMD), which improves after androgen replacement [47, 50]. Concerning the effects of hormone replacement over the increase of the bone mineral density, it was demonstrated that the use of testosterone isolated or associated with finasteride presented similar results, with the improvement of BMD in addition to the reduction of deoxypyridinoline, a urinary marker of bone absorption. This improvement was accompanied by a lower increase in prostatic size and absence of alterations in the PSA levels in patients who used the testosterone associated with the finasteride [50]. Still in relation to the bone density, an association was found between the levels of estrogens, in men, and bone density, suggesting that estrogens are beneficial to the maintenance of BMD on both women and men [47, 52]. Another aspect strongly related to low testosterone levels is the reduction in physical strength. Many studies found reduction in the physical strength on muscles of the superior and/or inferior parts of the body, while some studies demonstrated an improvement in physical strength after testosterone replacement therapy [47, 53]. An aggravation in the physical functioning aspects of these patients with significant improvement after the hormonal replacement therapy has also been pointed out [47, 48, 53]. The improvement in strength and physical functioning was also presented in patients treated with testosterone associated with finasteride [53]. Patients with reduction of bone mineral density secondary to hypogonadism present a disruption in many aspects analyzed by the QoL questionnaires, involving physical functioning, social functioning, and general health [54]. Crawford et al. (2003) demonstrated that the testosterone replacement promotes the improvement of the QoL alongside to the advancement of muscular mass and bone density [55].

The quality of the sexual life is an important aspect of QoL, having great psychological influence, constantly having to be researched and evaluated. The patients with hypogonadism present reduction of libido and increase in the sexual dysfunction rate with reduced frequency of spontaneous erections by morning in addition to difficulties in reaching and maintaining erection during sex [47]. The patients in hormonal replacement therapy mentioned improvement in sexual desire, quantity of sexual activity, in sexual satisfaction, and even ejaculation [48,56]. Patients with hypogonadism secondary to prostate cancer present alterations of QoL similar to elderly patients with hypogonadism, such as reduction in physical and functional well-being, rise of concerns, and aggravation in the sexual function [57]. Patients with hypogonadism and erectile dysfunction present reduction of the physical, psychological, environmental and social relations domains [58].

Another important finding in these patients is the association between the reduction of the serum levels of bioavailable testosterone and rise of depressive humor. This association was independent of age, weight variations, and physical activity [59]. In the A-RHDQoL specific questionnaire, the main domains under negative influence of the hormonal reduction were memory, energy, sexual life, and physical vigor [46].

An important relation pointed by some studies is the one between the fall of testosterone levels and glucose intolerance. In a large populational study, lower levels of total testosterone were found in men with reduction of glucose tolerance, elevated post prandial glycemia, or Diabetes Mellitus type 2, with this relation being kept even after adjusts for the body mass index [60]. In another study, prospective this time, an association between lower levels of testosterone in men and a higher chance of developing Diabetes Mellitus type 2 was demonstrated [61]. Costa Jr et al. (2011) revealed that the presence of Diabetes Mellitus implies in significant reduction in the QoL, nevertheless, more studies are necessary to associate androgenic replacement with the improvement in the QoL related to adequate glycemic control [62]. These alterations point towards the necessity of multiprofessional health teams, essential for the reaching of desired glycemic levels

All these alterations related to hypogonadism have great negative influence in the QoL of elderly men, which must be closely followed-up by specialists. However, the resistance presented by men in looking for medical help may be a drawback in the treatment of these patients, prolonging their suffering and making necessary the creation of campaigns and actions that promote a larger concern by the masculine population with their own health.

Conclusion

The hypogonadism is a condition of extreme importance because it can be experienced by people during the most different phases of life. Among its consequences, we draw attention to the commitment of the QoL. The elderly are the most affected patients, deserving special attention since besides the hypogonadism deleterious effects, they usually present reduction in the QoL secondary to their own age or to other comorbidities prevalent in the elderly population.

The health professionals must be prepared to recognize and treat the hypogonadism satisfactorily in both sexes during all phases of life of a person. Multiprofessional teams with good integration between its members must be developed for the treatment of these patients, aiming at a better approach to the signals and symptoms, which are extremely varied. In these patients, psychological and emotional questions are also very important independently of the age, with the necessity of psychological support by qualified professionals all the time, which is many times forgotten in the medical approach of patients with hypogonadism.

Despite the great changes that hypogonadism causes in the life of an individual, it is possible for these people to present a normal life. And, only with the union between patient, family, health professionals, friends, and the whole society will we be able to overcome the barriers that still exist and allow these people to no longer feel different and excluded.

References

[1] Cruz T. P., Pontes L., Vilar L. Hipogonadismo masculino. In: Vilar L.; Kater C. E., Naves L. A., Freitas M. C., Bruno O. D. (ed). *Endocrinologia Clínica.* 4th ed. Rio de Janeiro, Brazil: Guanabara Koogan; 2009:509-529.

[2] Costa E. M. F., Latronico A. C., Mendonça B. B. Retardo Puberal – Avaliação e Manuseio. In: Vilar L., Kater C. E., Naves L. A., Freitas M. C., Bruno O. D. (ed) *Endocrinologia Clínica.* 4th ed. Rio de Janeiro: Guanabara Koogan; 2009:213-227.

[3] Seftel A. D. Male hypogonadism. Part I: Epidemiology of hypogonadism. *Int J Impot Res.,* 2006, 18:115–120.

[4] Lee P., Ho K. K.Y. Hypopituitarism and Groth Hormone Deficiency. In: Jameson, J. Larry; DeGroot, Leslie J, editors. *Endocrinology.* 6th ed. Philadelphia: W. B. Saunders Company; 2010:243-261.

[5] Spritzer P. M., Mallmann E. S., Vilar L. Abordagem Diagnóstico-terapêutica da Amenorréia. Vilar L.; Kater C. E., Naves L. A., Freitas M. C., Bruno O. D. (ed). *Endocrinologia Clínica.* 4th ed. Rio de Janeiro: Guanabara Koogan; 2009:564-573.

[6] De Pergola G., De Mitrio V., Sciaraffia M., Pannacciulli N., Minenna A., Giorgino F., et al. Lower androgenicity is associated with higher plasma levels of prothrombotic factors irrespective of age, obesity, body fat distribution, and related metabolic parameters in men. *Metabolism,* 1997, 46(11):1287-1293.

[7] Hak A. E., Witteman J.C., de Jong F. H., Geerlings M. I., Hofman A., Pols H. A. Low levels of endogenous androgens increase the risk of atherosclerosis in elderly men: The Rotterdam Study. *J Clin Endocrinol Metab.,* 2002, 87(8):3632-3639.

[8] Barnhart K. T., Freeman E., Grisso J. A., Rader D. J., Sammel M., Kapoor S., et al. The effect of dehydroepiandrosterone supplementation to symptomatic perimenopausal women on serum endocrine profiles, lipid parameters, and health-related quality of life. *J Clin Endocrinol Metab.,* 1999, 84(11):3896-3902.

[9] Davison S., Davis S. New markers for cardiovascular disease risk in women: Impact of endogenous estrogen status and exogenous

postmenopausal hormone therapy. *J Clin Endocrinol Metab*., 2003, 88:2470-2478.

[10] Rexrode K. M., Manson J.E., Lee I. M., Ridker P. M., Sluss P. M., Cook N. R., et al. Sex hormone levels and risk of cardiovascular events in postmenopausal women. *Circulation*., 2003, 108(14):1688-1693.

[11] Braucks G. R., Naliato E. C. O., Tabet A. L., Gadelha M. R., Violante A. H. D. Clinical and therapeutic aspects of prolactinoma in men. *Arq Neuropsiquiatr*., 2003, 61(4):1004-1010.

[12] Melmed S., Kleinberg D. Anterior Pituitary. In: Larsen P. R., Kronenberg H. M., Melmed S., Polonsky K. S. (ed). *Williams Textbook of Endocrinology*. 10th ed. Philadelphia: W. B. Saunders Company; 2002:177-279.

[13] Grumbach M. M., Styne D. M. Puberty: Ontogeny, Neuroendocrinology, Physiology, and Disorders. In: Larsen P. R., Kronenberg H. M., Melmed S., Polonsky K. S. (ed). *Williams Textbook of Endocrinology*. 10th ed. Philadelphia: W. B. Saunders Company; 2002:1115-1286.

[14] Dobs A. S., Nguyen T., Pace C., Roberts C. P. Differential effects of oral estrogen *versus* oral estrogen-androgen replacement therapy on body composition in postmenopausal women. *J Clin Endocrinol Metab*., 2002, 87(4):1509-1516.

[15] Sherwin B. B. Estrogen and/or androgen replacement therapy and cognitive functioning in surgically menopausal women. *Psychoneuroendocrinology*, 1988, 13(4):345-357.

[16] Grady D., Herrington D., Bittner V., Blumenthal R., Davidson M., Hlatky M. et al. Cardiovascular disease outcomes during 6.8 years of hormone therapy - Heart and Estrogen/Progestin Replacement study follow-up (HERS II). *JAMA*, 2002, 288(1):49-57.

[17] Luyer M. D., Khosla S., Owen W. G., Miller V. M. Prospective randomized study of effects of unopposed estrogen replacement therapy on markers of coagulation and inflammation in postmenopausal women. *J Clin Endocrinol Metab*., 2001, 86(8):3629-3634.

[18] Majmudar N. G., Robson S. C., Ford G. A. Effects of the menopause, gender, and estrogen replacement therapy on vascular nitric oxide activity. *J Clin Endocrinol Metab*., 2000, 85(4):1577-1583.

[19] Brawer M. K. Androgen Supplementation and Prostate Cancer Risk: Strategies for Pretherapy Assessment and Monitoring. *Rev Urol.*, 2003, 5 (Suppl 1):S29-33.

[20] Steinberg K. K., Thacker S. B., Smith S. J., Stroup D. F., Zack M. M., Flanders W. D., et al. A meta-analysis of the effect of Estrogen Replacement Therapy on the Risk of Breast Cancer. *JAMA,* 1991, 265(15):1985-1990.

[21] Pike M. C., Peters R. K., Cozen W., Probst-Hensch N. M., Felix J. C., Wan P. C., et al. Estrogen-Progestin Replacement Therapy and Endometrial Cancer. *J Natl Cancer Inst.*, 1997, 89(15):1110-1116.

[22] WHOQOL Group. The World Health Organization quality of life assessment (WHOQOL): Position paper from the World Health Organization. *Soc Sci Med.*, 1995, 41(10):1403-1409.

[23] Carel J. C., Ecosse E., Bastie-Sigeac I., Cabrol S., Tauber M., Léger J., et al. Quality of Life Determinants in Young Women with Turner's Syndrome after Growth Hormone Treatment: Results of the StaTur Population-Based Cohort Study. *J Clin Endocrinol Metab.*, 2005, 90(4):1992-1997.

[24] Amundson E., Boman U. W., Barrenäs M. L., Bryman I., Landin-Wilhelmsen K., et al. . Impact of Growth Hormone Therapy on Quality of Life in Adults with Turner Syndrome. *J Clin Endocrinol Metab.*, 2010, 95(3):1355-1359.

[25] Sutton E.J., McInerney-Leo A.,; Bondy C. A., Gollust S. E., King D., Biesecker B., et al. Turner Syndrome: Four Challenger Across the Lifespan. *Am J Med Genet A.*, 2005, 139A(2):57-66.

[26] Okada Y. The Quality of Life of Turner Women in Comparison with Grown-Up GH-Deficient Women. *Endocr J.*, 1994, 41(4):345-354.

[27] Carel J. C., Elie C., Ecosse E., Tauber M., Léger J., Cabrol S., et al. Self-Esteem and Social Adjustment in Young Women with Turner Syndrome—Influence of Pubertal Management and Sexuality: Population-Based Cohort Study. *J Clin Endocrinol Metab.*, 2006, 91(8):2972-2979.

[28] Johannsen T. H., Ripa C. P., Mortensen E. L., Main K. M. Quality of life in 70 women with disorders of sex development. *Eur J Endocrinol.*, 2006, 155(6):877-885.

[29] de Ronde W., de Haan A., Drent M. L. Quality of life is reduced in patients with Klinefelter syndrome on androgen replacement therapy. *Eur J Endocrinol.*, 2009, 160(3):465-468.

[30] Ratcliffe S. Long term outcome in children of sex chromosome abnormalities. *Arch Dis Chil.,* 1999, 80:192-195.

[31] Rovet J., Netley C., Keenan M., Bailey J., Stewart D. The Psychoeducational Profile of Boys with Klinefelter Syndrome. *J Learn Disabil.*, 1996, 29(2):180-196.

[32] Bruining H., Swaab H., Kas M., van Engeland H. Psychiatric Characteristics in a Self-Selected Sample of Boys With Klinefelter Syndrome. *Pediatrics*, 2009, 123(5):e865-870.

[33] Corona G., Petrone L., Paggi F., Lotti F., Boddi V., Fisher A., et al. Sexual dysfunction in subjects with Klinefelter's syndrome. *Int J Androl.*, 2010,33(4):574-580.

[34] Jackson S., Morris M. Appearance Matters: the impact of perceived altered appearance as a result of Klinefelter's Syndrome on psycho-social functioning. Presented at 11th European Congress of Endocrinology, Istanbul, Turkey. *Endocrine Abstracts **20** OC6.4.*

[35] Hilditch J. R., Lewis J., Peter A., van Maris B., Ross A., Franssen E., et al. A menopause-specific quality of life questionnaire: development and psychometric properties. *Maturitas,* 1996, 24(3):161-175.

[36] Rahman S., Salehin F., Iqbal A. Menopausal symptoms assessment among middle age women in Kushtia, Bangladesh. *BMC Res Notes*, 2011, 4:188-191.

[37] Im E.O., Lee B., Chee W., Brown A., Dormire S. Menopausal Symptoms Among Four Major Ethnic Groups in the U.S. *West J Nurs Res.*, 2010, 32(4):540-565.

[38] Chuni N., Sreeramareddy C. T. Frequency of symptoms, determinants of severe symptoms, validity of and cut-off score for Menopause Rating Scale (MRS) as a screening tool: A cross-sectional survey among midlife Nepalese women. *BMC Womens Health*, 2011, 11:30-38.

[39] Ohayon M. M. Severe Hot Flashes Are Associated With Chronic Insomnia. *Arch Intern Med.*, 2006, 166(12):1262-1268.

[40] Huang A. J., Subak L. L., Wing R., West D. S., Hernandez A. L., Macer J., et al. An Intensive Behavioral Weight Loss Intervention and Hot Flushes in Women. *Arch Intern Med.*, 2010, 170(13):1161-1167.

[41] Tranah G. J., Parimi N., Blackwell T., Ancoli-Israel S., Ensrud K. E., Cauley J. A., et al. Post menopausal hormones and sleep quality in the elderly: a population based study. *BMC Womens Health*, 2010, 10:15.

[42] Huang A. J., Luft J., Grady D., Kuppermann M. The Day-to-Day Impact of Urogenital Aging: Perspectives from Racially/Ethnically Diverse Women. *J Gen Intern Med.*, 2010, 25(1):45-51.

[43] Huang A. J., Moore E. E., Boyko E. J., Scholes D., Lin F., Vittinghoff E., et al. Vaginal symptoms in postmenopausal women: self-reported

severity, natural history, and risk factors. *Menopause*, 2010, 17(1):121-126.

[44] Ağıl A., Abıke F., Daşkapan A., Alaca R., Tüzün H. Short-Term Exercise Approaches on Menopausal Symptoms, Psychological Health, and Quality of Life in Postmenopausal Women. *Obstet Gynecol Int.*, 2010, 2010. pii: 274261.

[45] Forouhari S., Khajehei M., Moattari M., Mohit M., Rad M. S., Ghaem H. The Effect of Education and Awareness on the Quality-of-Life in Postmenopausal Women. *Indian J Community Med.*, 2010, 35(1):109-114.

[46] McMillan C. V., Bradley C., Giannoulis M., Martin F., Sönksen P. H. Preliminary development of a new individualized questionnaire measuring quality of life in older men with age related hormonal decline: the A-RHDQoL. *Health Qual Life Outcomes.*, 2003, 1:51.

[47] Basaria S., Lieb 2nd J., Tang A. M., DeWeese T., Carducci M., Eisenberger M., et al. Long-term effects of androgen deprivation therapy in prostate cancer patients. *Clin Endocrinol. (Oxf)*, 2002, 56(6):779-786.

[48] Fennell C., Sartorius G., Ly L. P., Turner L., Liu P. Y., Conway A.J., et al. Randomized cross-over clinical trial of injectable vs. implantable depot testosterone for maintenance of testosterone replacement therapy in androgen deficient men. *Clin Endocrinol. (Oxf)*, 2010, 73(1):102-109.

[49] Ly L. P., Jimenez M., Zhuang T. N., Celermajer D. S., Conway A. J., Handelsman D. J. A Double-Blind, Placebo-Controlled, Randomized Clinical Trial of Transdermal Dihydrotestosterone Gel on Muscular Strength, Mobility, and Quality of Life in Older Men with Partial Androgen Deficiency. *J Clin Endocrinol Metab.*, 2001, 86(9):4078-4088.

[50] Amory, JK; Watts, NB; Easley, KA; Sutton, PR; Anawalt, BD; Matsumoto, AM; et al. Exogenous Testosterone or Testosterone with Finasteride Increases Bone Mineral Density in Older Men with Low Serum Testosterone. *J Clin Endocrinol Metab.*, 2004; 89(2):503-10.

[51] Thein M., Ershler W. B., Artz A. S., Tecson J., Robinson B. E., Rothstein G., et al. Diminished Quality of Life and Physical Function in Community-Dwelling Elderly with Anemia. *Medicine (Baltimore),* 2009, 88(2):107-114.

[52] Naliato E. C. O., Farias M. L., Braucks G. R., Costa F. S., Zylberberg D., Violante A. H. D. Prevalence of osteopenia in men with prolactinoma. *J Endocrinol Invest*., 2005, 28(1):12-17.

[53] Page S. T., Amory J. K., Bowman F. D., Anawalt B. D., Matsumoto A. M., Bremner W. J., et al. Exogenous Testosterone (T) Alone or with Finasteride Increases Physical Performance, Grip Strength, and Lean Body Mass in Older Men with Low Serum T. *J Clin Endocrinol Metab*., 2005, 90(3):1502-1510.

[54] Dennison E. M., Jameson K. A., Syddall H. E., Martin H. J., Cushnaghan J., Aihie S. A., et al. Bone health and deterioration in quality of life among participants from the Hertfordshire cohort study. *Osteoporos Int*., 2010, 21(11):1817-1824.

[55] Crawford B. A., Liu P. Y., Kean M. T., Bleasel J. F., Handelsman D. J. Randomized Placebo-Controlled Trial of Androgen Effects on Muscle and Bone in Men Requiring Long- Term Systemic Glucocorticoid Treatment. *J Clin Endocrinol Metab*., 2003, 88(7):3167-3176.

[56] Greenfield D. M., Walters S. J., Coleman R. E., Hancock B. W., Snowden J. A., Shalet S. M., et al. Quality of Life, Self-Esteem, Fatigue, and Sexual Function in Young Men After Cancer. *Cancer*, 2010, 116(6):1592-1601.

[57] Fleishman S. B., Khan H., Homel P., Suhail M. F., Strebel-Amrhein R., Mohammad F., et al. Testosterone Levels and Quality of Life in Diverse Male Patients With Cancers Unrelated to Androgens. *J Clin Oncol*., 2010, 28(34):5054-5060.

[58] Hwang T. I., Lo H. C., Tsai T. F., Chiou H. Y. Association among hypogonadism, quality of life and erectile dysfunction in middle-aged and aged male in Taiwan. *Int J Impot Res*., 2007, 19(1):69-75.

[59] Barrett-Connor E., Von Mühlen D. G., Kritz-Silverstein D. Bioavailable Testosterone and Depressed Mood in Older Men: The Rancho Bernardo Study. *J Clin Endocrinol Metab*., 1999, 84(2):573-577.

[60] Goodman-Gruen, D; Barrett-Connor, E. Sex Differences in the Association of Endogenous Sex Hormone Levels and Glucose Tolerance Status in Older Men and Women. *Diabetes Care*, 2000, 23(7):912-918.

[61] Oh J. Y., Barrett-Connor E., Wedick N. M., Wingard D. L. Rancho Bernardo Study. Endogenous Sex Hormones and the Development of Type 2 Diabetes in Older Men and Women: the Rancho Bernardo Study. *Diabetes Care*, 2002, 25(1):55-60.

[62] Costa Jr, A. C., Miranda M. P., Moura J. C., Martins C. F., Oliveira P. S., Cerqueira E. F. S., et al. Diabetes Mellitus and Quality of Life in Hospitalized Patients. *Endocr Rev.,* 2011; 32: P1-526.

In: Quality of Life in Endocrine Diseases ISBN: 978-1-63463-911-8
Editor: Erika Cesar de Oliveira Naliato © 2015 Nova Science Publishers, Inc.

Chapter 7

Quality of Life in Hyper- and Hypothyroidism

Vinicius C. Mota, Minelli S. A. Fernandes, Nichole V. C. R. Coutinho and Erika C. O. Naliato*

Center of Studies Ricardo A T Castilho of the Teresópolis Medical Association, Brazil

Abbreviations

ATD	anti-thyroid drugs
D1	deiodinase type 1
D2	deiodinase type 2
GD	Graves' Disease
HCG	human chorionic gonadotropin
HLA-B8	human leukocyte antigen B8
PTU	propylthiouracil
QoL	quality of life
T3	triiodothyronine
T4	thyroxine
TA	toxic adenoma
TMG	toxic multinodular goiter

* Correspondence to: erikanaliato@uol.com.br.

TRAb	TSH-receptor antibodies
TSH	thyroid-stimulating hormone / thyrotropic hormone
TSHoma	TSH-producing pituitary adenoma
WHO	World Health Organization

Introduction

Thyroid dysfunction is a common disease. In the United States, hypothyroidism is present in 4.6% of the population, where 0.3% present clinical hypothyroidism and 4.3% subclinical hypothyroidism [1]. In the United Kingdom, studies point out to an incidence of hyperthyroidism in 0.8% per 1000 women/year and of hypothyroidism in 3.5% per 1000 women/year [2]. Many factors are involved in the genesis of the thyroid dysfunctions which include the auto-immune mechanisms, genetic factors related to the HLA complex and environmental factors. The iodine nutritional deficiency is the most common cause of goiter in the world, which is a public health problem in 130 countries affecting 1.5 billion people or 13% of the world population [3]. The minimum recommended daily ingestion of iodine is 75 μg/day which corresponds to 10 g of iodized salt in accordance with the recommendations of the World Health Organization (one part of potassium iodine in 100.000 parts of NaCl) [4].

In humans, the thyroid synthetizes thyroid hormones in order to stimulate the development and growth of the diverse organs and systems. The main hormone produced by the thyroid is thyroxine (T4). Despite that, the triiodothyronine (T3) is the metabolically active hormone. In normal conditions, all the circulating T4 and 20% of T3 are directly produced by the thyroid, the other 80% result from the deiodination of T4 in peripheral tissues through the action of the deiodinase type 1 (D1) and type 2 (D2). In general lines, the thyroid function is regulated by the thyrotropin-releasing hormone which through the hypothalamic-pituitary portal system is directed to the anterior pituitary linking itself to specific receptors of the thyrotroph and inducing the synthesis and secretion of the thyroid-stimulating hormone / thyrotropic hormone (TSH). This, in turn, interacts with the receptors present in the thyroid follicular cell membrane inducing the expression of proteins involved in the biosynthesis of thyroid hormones, increasing the thyroid cell activity and stimulating hormone secretion [5]. The values of the produced hormones give us parameters and are fundamental for the diagnosis of the possible pathologies as observed in Table 1 [6].

Table 1. Interpretation of Thyroid function

	High T4	Normal T4	Low T4
High TSH	In vivo or in vitro artefact Pituitary hyperthyroidism [TSHoma] Thyroid hormone resistance	Mild thyroid failure (primary) (also termed subclinical hypothyroidism And diminished thyroid reserve)	Primary Hypotireoidism
Normal TSH	As above Sampling within 6 h of thyroxine dose	Normal (in patients taking thyroxine, TSH > 3mU/L may indicate subtle underreplacement)	Hypothalamic or pituitary Hypothyroidism Severe non-thyroidian accute disease
Low TSH	Hypertireoidism (for this diagnosis, TSH must be suppressed rather than just low)	Subclinical hyperthyroidism Subtle thyroxine overreplacement Thyroid autonomy (multinodular goitre or autonomous functioning thyroid nodule) Non-thyroidal illness	Hypothalamic or pituitary Hypothyroidism Severe non-thyroidian accute disease

Adapted from Stockigt (2001).

Hypotiroidism

Hypothyroidism is the most common cause of pathological hormone deficiency presenting an ample gamma of clinical manifestations which vary from an asymptomatic state to coma, with multiple failures of organs and systems [7]. Its presentation involves as the most remarkable manifestations: asthenia, somnolence, cold intolerance, dry and flaky skin, slurred voice, deep hyporeflexia, facial edema, anemia and bradycardia. The syndrome globally compromises the organism, hence the variety of the symptomatology with which the syndrome may express itself. Despite that, many patients may be asymptomatic or oligosymptomatic. This happens mostly in those with less intense or short-length disease [8]. Occasionally, patients may present just paresthesia in arms and legs [9]. The complete expression of the hypothyroidism is known as myxedema [8].

More frequently (90-95% of the cases), it reflects an abnormality of the thyroid gland itself (primary hypothyroidism); however, it may be caused by pituitary disease (secondary hypothyroidism) or hypothalamic disease (tertiary hypothyroidism), where these latter can be named central hypothyroidism since the distinction between the pituitary and hypothalamic is not always possible to be achieved [10]. The etiologies are diverse, as seen in Table 2, but in adults, the most frequent cause is the auto-immune disease, the main example being Hashimoto disease or chronic lymphocytic thyroiditis [7].

Table 2. Etiology of hypothyroidism

Primary hypothyroidism:
Reduction of the thyroid functioning tissue:
- Hashimoto thyroiditis
- Subacute (granulomatous and lymphocytic) thyroiditis
- Postpartum thyroiditis
- Riedel thyroiditis
- Graves' Disease and treatment of hyperthyroidism
- Infiltrative diseases (amyloidosis, hemochromatosis, cystinosis, progressive systemic sclerosis, sarcoidosis)
- Thyroid agenesis and ectopias
- Head, neck and whole body external radiotherapy
Functional defects of the biosynthesis and liberation of thyroid hormones:
- Congenital dyshormonogenesis
- Severe iodine deficiency
- Drugs (anti-thyroid, iodine, lithium, amiodarone, radiology contrasts, sodium valproate, sunitinib, synthetic or natural goiter drugs, etc.)

Central hypothyroidism:
Loss of functioning tissue:
- Tumors (pituitary adenoma, craniopharyngioma, meningioma, dysgerminoma, glioma, metastases)
- Trauma (surgery, radiotherapy, cranial trauma)
- Vascular (Sheehan syndrome, pituitary apoplexy, stem section, internal carotid aneurysm)
- Infections (abscess, tuberculosis, syphilis, toxoplasmosis)
- Infiltrative diseases (sarcoidosis, histiocytosis, hemochromatosis)
- Chronic lymphocytic hypophysitis
- Congenital lesions (pituitary hypoplasia, septooptic dysplasia, basal encephalocele)
Functional defects of the biosynthesis and liberation of TSH:
- Mutations on the genes of TSH and TRH receptors, or TSH-ß, POU1F1, PROP1 e HESX1 genes - Drugs (dopamine, dobutamine, glycocorticoids, bexarotene, interruption of therapy with L-thyroxine)

Hashimoto disease constitutes the most prevalent form of thyroid autoimmune disease, being three times more common in women and has its diagnosis more frequently made between the third and fifth decades of life. The genetic tendency of the disease is demonstrated by a familiar incidence rise and by an association with major histocompatibility antigens, such as HLA-B8. The presence of antiperoxidase antibodies (in 95% of the cases) and antithyroglobulin (60% of the cases) indicates the autoimmune nature of the disease [10]. Patients with autoimmune thyroiditis may vary from hypothyroidism and euthyroidism, to transient thyrotoxicosis conditions followed by hypothyroidism (Hashitoxicosis) [7].

The treatment indicated for hypothyroidism consists in the hormonal replacement with sodium levothyroxine for which there are many commercial names; however, it is recommended to keep the patient with the same commercial presentation, at least during the period of dose adjustment [11]. The dose in young adults may vary between 1.2 to 1.7 μg/kg/day and, in elderly patients, between 1 to 1.5 μg/kg/day, where the average replacement dose is around 112 and 119 μg/day [12]. The etiology of the hypothyroidism may influence the value of the required levothyroxine dose. Patients whose hypothyroidism is a result of autoimmune chronic thyroiditis, total and gestational thyroidectomy may need higher doses of levothyroxine. As a result, the initial dose of levothyroxine may vary considerable in the same patient or between different patients as a function of age, weight, cardiac condition, severity and length of hypothyroidism [13]. In particular, geriatric patients and those with history of cardiovascular disease are recommended to start the treatment slower with doses of 12.5-25.0 μg/day for 3-4 weeks, increasing in 25 μg every four weeks until reaching the sufficient dose for the normalization of the TSH [12].

Hyperthyroidism

The hyperthyroidism is a pathological syndrome in which the tissues are exposed to excessive quantities of thyroid hormone and has as main causes Graves' Disease (GD), followed by toxic multinodular goiter (TMG) and toxic adenoma (TA). Table 3 shows the different etiologies of the disease [14].

Table 3. Etiology of Hyperthyroidism

Dependent on the increased production of thyroid hormone: Abnormal stimulation of the thyroid by thyroid-stimulating immunoglobulins - Graves' Disease - Hashimoto's Thyroiditis Abnormal stimulation of the thyroid by human chorionic gonadotropin (hCG): - Hydatiform mole - Choriocarcinoma Excessive production of TSH: - TSHomas - Pituitary resistance to T3 and T4 Excessive autonomous production of T3 and T4 (independent of TSH): - Toxic adenoma (mutation of TSH receptor) - Toxic multinodular goiter - Follicular carcinoma - Jod-Basedow phenomenon (excess of amiodarone or iodine-induced hypothyroidism)
Independent of increased production of thyroid hormone: Increased release of T3 and T4: - Subacute granulomatous thyroiditis (painful) - Subacute lymphocytic thyroiditis (not painful) Extra-thyroid source - Factitious thyrotoxicosis - Hamburger thyrotoxicosis Ectopic production of T3 and T4 - ovarian teratoma (struma ovarii) - Functioning metastasis of the follicular carcinoma

The clinical manifestations are a result of the stimulatory effect of the thyroid hormones over the metabolism and tissues. Among the most characteristics are nervousness, insomnia, weight loss (despite polyphagia), tachycardia, palpitations, heat intolerance, excessive perspiration with hot and humid skin, tremors, muscular weakness and hyper-defecation [15]. A comparison between the main manifestations of hypo and hyperthyroidism is shown in Table 4.

GD is an autoimmune disease characterized by the presence of autoantibodies directly against the TSH receptor. Some of these antibodies (TRAb) mimic the effects of the pituitary TSH, stimulating the growth and the function of the thyroid gland, being present in more than 90% of the cases. Other autoantibodies, such as the antinuclear factor, antiperoxidase and antithyroglobulin may also be found elevated. GD affects women more than men (8:1) and the appearance of symptoms usually occurs between the 20 and 40 years of age. The thyroid gland is found diffusely enlarged, symmetric and with prominent vascularization. It may be accompanied by infiltrative ophthalmopathy (exophthalmia) in 30% of the cases, and less frequently, by infiltrative dermopathy (pretibial myxedema) [16].

Table 4. Main signs and symptoms of the hypothyroidism X hyperthyroidism

	Hypothyroidism	**Hyperthyroidism**
Behavior	Mental slowness Quietness Somnolence Sensibility to cold	Mental quickness Restlessness Excitability Sensibility to heat
Organism	Deficient growth or + nitrogen balance Low basal metabolism Hypercholesterolemia Myxedema	Excessive growth or - nitrogen balance High basal metabolism Hypocholesterolemia Exophthalmia
Cardiovascular system	Bradycardia Decrease of circulatory speed Slow pulse	Tachycardia, palpitations Increase of circulatory speed Fast pulse
Gastrointestinal system	Hypophagia Constipation Decreased glucose uptake	Hyperphagia Diarrhea Increased glucose uptake
Muscle	Hypotonia Muscle weakness	Fibrillation, tremors Muscle weakness
Immune mechanisms	Susceptibility to infections	Susceptibility to infections
Tissues	Low O_2 consumption	High O_2 consumption
Enzymes	Decrease of oxidative enzymes	Increase of oxidative enzymes

The development of one or more autonomous thyroid nodules which produce excessive quantity of thyroid hormone is also a common dysfunction. Its frequency increases with age and it is more common in women. There are no antibodies directed against the TSH receptor or the anti-peroxidase, which are present in GD [14].

Initial treatment for GD is established with anti-thyroid drugs (ATD). Definitive treatment is performed with surgery (thyroidectomy) or ^{131}I. Beta-blockers may be used in order to decrease adrenergic signs. ATD inhibit T3 and T4 synthesis and act on the immune system; propylthiouracil (PTU) also decreases the peripheral conversion of T4 to T3. PTU is recommended in 5-10mg/kg/day; metimazol, in 0.5-1.0mg/kg/day. L-tiroxine (100μg/m²/day) should be added when euthyroidism is obtained. The remission rate is low. Adverse effects such as skin rash, nausea, headache, and arthralgia are frequent, while hepatitis, vasculitis, purpura and agranulocytosis are rare. Relapse may be conducted with another cycle of ATD, thyroidectomy or ^{131}I. Mortality is low in those submitted to surgical treatment (0.08%) and the cure index reaches 80%. ^{131}I is safer and cost-effective and has been used more frequently as a first option for definitive therapy in many countries. Elevated doses are used to reach complete ablation of the thyroid gland. Post-surgery or iodine hypothyroidism must be adequately treated with L-thyroxine. Both surgery and radioiodine treatment are indicated in hyperthyroidism secondary to mutations in the TSH-receptor or G-protein alpha-subunit genes. Surgery is the best option for TSH-producing tumors. In the thyroid hormone resistance syndrome, T3 or tri-iodinated tyro-ascetic acid has been used. Follicular rupture-induced hyperthyroidism is managed solely with beta-blockers [17].

The symptoms of these thyroid dysfunctions are sometimes varied and unspecific and are frequently found in the general population even without the presence of specific dysfunctions, which makes the diagnosis even harder to be established and clinical management tends to be delayed [18]. Therefore, the clinical manifestations of the above mentioned diseases may compromise the quality of life (QoL). In addition, dissatisfaction with treatment due to persistence of symptoms has been reported [19, 20]. In conclusion, it is important to evaluate and monitor QoL in patients with thyroid diseases.

Quality of Life in Patients with Thyroid Disease

QoL is an outcome measure that has been enthusiastically used by clinicians, researchers, economists, administrators and politicians. Although the concept of QoL is not new, its importance has been growing for a number of reasons. In 1948, the World Health Organization (WHO) defined Health not only as the absence of disease, but also as the presence of physical, mental, and social well-being. Recently, QoL has been reinforced as a necessary concept in the practice of care and research in the Health field [21]. In order to directly measure individual health, some structured and simplified instruments, able to recognize states of complete physical, mental and social well-being, have been developed and tested [22]. QoL is an important measure of the impact on health [23, 24]. The interest for the measurement of QoL is relatively recent, either in the fields of disease prevention or health promotion [25] and its evaluation seems important in the case of hyper- and hypothyroidism, since the symptoms and signs can strongly impair patients' life.

The understanding of QoL throughout the years has led to the valorization of both objective and subjective aspects. There is no consensus about its concept, but the aspects of subjectiveness and multidimensionality are usually accepted by the majority of researchers [26].

Studies of QoL in patients with thyroid diseases are limited by the fact that the duration of hyper- and hypothyroidism is frequently unknown by a significant portion of the patients. In patients with subclinical hyperthyroidism, QoL is usually preserved and the restauration of euthyroidism does not seem to affect QoL in this subset of patients [27].

The role of hormonal alterations and comorbidities of thyroid diseases in the impairment of QoL has been questioned. It seems that the persistent impairment of QoL is very frequent is thyroid diseases such as hyper- and hypothyroidism. However, due to the broad clinical spectrum of hypothyroidism, QoL evaluation is difficult in this group, when compared to hyperthyroidism [28].

Patients with non-treated thyroid disease suffer from a variety of symptoms and present impairment in the majority of QoL questionnaires. For instance, 22 to 35% of the patients with goiter, 18 to 66% of those with hyperthyroidism, and 7 to 99% of those with ophthalmopathy experience limitation to perform daily activities when in treatment for the respective diseases. These prevalence intervals are broad due to the use of different forms of measurement of the concepts, variety of populations interviewed, and diversity of question categorization. However, there is evidence of impairment in all groups. In patients with goiter, hyperthyroidism, and ophthalmopathy, it becomes evident throughout the low punctuation in general health perception scales, compared to normal controls. Nevertheless, 53 to 100% of patients classified their health as impaired.

Therefore, a substantial proportion of patients with thyroid diseases experiences limitations in their daily activities, perceive their general health as impaired and detect emotional and social impairment. Cognitive problems are also common [29].

Recent studies have not detected correlations between TSH levels and QoL in patients with hyperthyroidism. Similarly, no study has clarified if there is a causal relationship between hyperthyroidism and cognitive decline, or if the association between low levels of TSH and dementia is influenced by an increased prevalence of non-thyroid disease in the elderly [30].

The relationship between the presence of symptoms of hypo- or hyperthyroidism and QoL has not been evaluated in long-term basis in follow-up studies of patients [29]. Nevertheless, results indicate an association between hypothyroidism and clinical features and symptoms of depression and anxiety, independently of the cause of hypothyroidism. It is estimated that 17% of patients with mood disturbances have hypothyroidism. In addition, symptoms of depression and anxiety have been demonstrated to increase with the elevation of serum levels of TSH [31]. Both hypo- and hyperthyroidism have been associated with symptoms such as fatigue, and disturbance of appetite and sleep, which impair the differential diagnosis with depression.

Low levels of thyroid hormones and high levels of TSH are associated with a delay in the therapeutic response in bipolar depression [32]. Dysregulation of thyroid function strongly affects the response to anti-depressive drugs. It is important to point out that depressive syndromes are common in a number of chronic diseases, and this can lead to lower adherence to treatment, worse clinical evolution, worse QoL, and higher morbidity and mortality. Considering these aspects, it is mostly important to treat depression as comorbidity, although there is a lack of studies to indicate the consequences of depression control in the evolution of chronic diseases [33].

Treatment of patients resistant to anti-depressive drugs with high doses of T3 showed improvement in 84% and remission in 33% of patients. Nevertheless, the use of thyroid hormones in order to treat depressive symptoms in individuals with subclinical hypothyroidism has not been proved effective until now [34].

A new instrument, the Underactive Thyroid-Dependent Quality of Life Questionnaire (ThyDQoL), has been created to assess the impact of hypothyroidism in different aspects of the patients' life. Furthermore, a new measure of symptoms of hypothyroidism, the Underactive Thyroid Symptom Rating Questionnaire (ThySRQ), evaluates the degree of disturbance induced by these symptoms. Both instruments have good sensibility, but so far still lack clinical assay application [35].

Cardiovascular effects of hyperthyroidism include the increase in cardiac frequency, with increased incidence of cardiac arrhythmias, and left ventricular hypertrophy. Patients with subclinical hyperthyroidism may experience signs and symptoms of adrenergic hyperactivity, particularly those younger than 50 years. Besides that, older patients with subclinical hyperthyroidism may be at risk for atrial fibrillation. These comorbidities may incur in impairment of QoL. In the only randomized prospective study to compare the three modalities of treatment for hyperthyroidism (pharmacological, surgical, and radioiodine), all of them resulted in QoL improvement [36-38].

Graves' ophthalmopathy may induce facial/orbital deformities and reduce visual capacity with significant impair of QoL [39, 40]. Moreover, the decline in physical function, mental health, and visual acuity may strongly influence daily activities, including social interaction [41]. As a consequence, Graves' ophthalmopathy has been linked with reduction of QoL, either in the physical and the emotional aspects [42-44].

The use of the presently available questionnaires limits the investigation of the impacts of Graves' Ophthalmopathy on psychological and emotional aspects. However, the quantitative approach permits the detailed exploration of patients and captures their experiences. Three main problems have been identified: (1) the development of an alteration of identity as a result of changes in appearance, ability and roles, due to the physical consequences of the ophthalmopathy; (2) development of strategies of contest and denial, including social abandonment, adjustment, and stoicism, and (3) difficult interaction with health professionals due to the uncertainty about choices, diagnosis, prognosis, and treatment, resulting in remoteness, anger, and frustration [40]. A quantitative study identified the existence of an identity alteration due to the direct consequences of Graves' Ophthalmopathy, which impact on the well-being, the coping strategies, and the interactions with health professionals. Treatment schemes for Graves' Ophthalmopathy are frequently of inferior quality, leaving patients with residual effects long after its completion.

Facial expressions and visual contact are essential components for communication. The fixed look sign observed in patients with Graves' Ophthalmopathy may be interpreted as hostile and evoke negative reactions from other people. These negative reactions and social stigmatization have been described in other conditions such as facial disfiguration, resulting frequently in social retreat [40].

The consequences of Graves' Ophthalmopathy and its treatment are in their majority evaluated by means of biological measures, such as the NOSPEC classification [45]. While biological measures are vital and produce valuable information for the physician, they are poorly correlated with the patients' personal experience regarding functional capacity and health perception [46].

Most authors agree that pharmacological treatment for Graves' Ophthalmopathy is effective in the acute phase of the disease, but the final results are frequently poor and a considerable portion of patients remains dissatisfied with their facial appearance. Nevertheless, there are still few studies on QoL in Graves' Ophthalmopathy [47, 48].

In the field of Ophthalmology, many instruments of self-evaluation of visual acuity have been developed since 1998. Three instruments – the ADVS (Activities of Daily Vision Scale), VFQ-25 (National Eye Institute Visual Function Questionnaire), and VF-14 (Visual Function Index) – have been largely used in patients with visual disturbances. Recently, the importance of the evaluation of visual acuity on QoL has been gaining progressive importance [41]. The first questionnaire for the evaluation of QoL in patients with ophthalmopathy has been developed [49]. This instrument measures limitations in the visual function as a consequence of diplopia and/or reduction in visual acuity (eight questions) and in psychosocial functioning as a modification of the appearance of the patient (eight questions). This questionnaire may be used in clinical studies to evaluate the influence of new modalities of treatment for ophthalmopathy [50, 51].

Conclusion

Thyroid disturbances are frequent, especially hypo- and hyperthyroidism. The diseases, when not properly diagnosed and treated, may lower QoL and impair adequate social and familiar interaction. Specific questionnaires, such as *ThyDQoL* and *ThySRQ* are being tested as instruments to measure patients' well-being and QoL.

References

[1] Hollowell J. G., Staehling N. W., Flanders W. D., et al. Serum TSH, T4 and thyroid antibodies in the United States population (1988-1994): National Health and Nutrition Survey (NHANES III). *J Clin Endocrinol Metab.,* 2002, 87:486-488.

[2] Vanderpump M. P., Tunbridge W. M., French J. M., et al. The incidence of thyroid disorders in the community: a twenty-year follow-up of the Whickham Survey. *Clin Endocrinol.,* 1995, 43:55-68.

[3] Pontes A. A, Adan L. F., Costa A. D. M., et al. Prevalência de doenças da tireóide em uma comunidade do Nordeste brasileiro. *Arq Bras Endocrinol Metab.*, 2002, 45:544-549.

[4] Dunn J.T. Endemic goiter and cretinism: an update on iodine status. *J Pediatr Endocrinol Metab.*, 2001, 14:1469-473.

[5] Greenspan F. S. The thyroid gland. In: Greenspan FS, Gardner DG (eds). *Basic & clinical endocrinology.* 7th ed. New York, USA: McGraw-Hill; 2004:215-294.

[6] Stockigt J. R. Free thyroid hormone measurement. A critical appraisal. *Endocrinol Metab Clin North Am.,* 2001, 30:265-289.

[7] Roberts C. G. P., Landenson P. W. Hypothyroidism. *Lancet,* 2004, 363:793-803.

[8] Danzig S., Klein I. Recent considerations in the treatment of hypothyroidism. *Curr Opin Investing Drugs,* 2008, 9:357-362.

[9] Marks P. W., Zukerberg L. R. Case records of the Massachussetts General Hospital. Weekly clinicopathological exercises. Case 30-2004. A 37-year-old woman with paresthesias of the arms and legs. *N Engl J Med.*, 2004, 351:1333-1341.

[10] Dillmann W. H. The thyroid. In: Goldman L, Ausiello, D. (eds) *Goldman's Cecil Medicine.* 22ª ed. Rio de Janeiro, Brazil: Elsevier; 2005:1617-1642.

[11] Briesacher B.A., Andrade S. E., Fouayzi H. Medication adherence and use of generic drug therapies. *Am J Manag Care*, 2009, 15:450-456.

[12] Fish L. H., Schwartz H.L., Cavanaugh J., et al. Replacement dose, metabolism, and bioavailability of levothyroxine in the treatment of hypothyroidism. Role of triiodothyronine in pituitary feedback in humans. *N Engl J Med.*, 1987, 316:764-770.

[13] Allahabadia A., Razvi S., Abraham P., et al. Diagnosis and treatment of primary hypothyroidism. *BMJ.,* 2009, 338:b725.

[14] Cooper D. S. Hyperthyroidism. *Lancet,* 2003, 362:459-468.

[15] Nayak B., Hodak S. P. Hyperthyroidism. *Endocrinol Metab Clin North Am.*, 2007, 36:617-656.

[16] Fritzgerald P. A. Disease of the thyroid gland. In: Tierney L. M., McPhee S. J., Papadakis M, A. (eds). *Current medical diagnosis & treatment.* 44th ed. New York, USA: Lange; 2005:1084-1112.

[17] Sandrini R., França S. N., Lacerda L., et al. Tratamento do hipertiroidismo na infância e adolescência. *Arq Bras Endocrinol Metab.,* 2001, 45(1):32-36.

[18] Ladenson P. W., Singer P. A., Ain K. B., et al. American Thyroid Association guidelines for detection of thyroid dysfunction. *Arch Intern Med.*, 2000, 160:1573–1575.

[19] *Roberts N. D. Psychological problems in thyroid disease. British Thyroid Foundation Newsletter.* 1996, *18*:3.

[20] Walsh J. P. Dissatisfaction with thyroxine therapy – could the patients be right? *Curr Opin Pharmacol.*, 2002, 2:717–722.

[21] Minayo M. C. S., Hartz Z. M. A., Buss P. M. Qualidade de vida e saúde: um debate necessário. *Ciencia Saúde Colet.,* 2000, 5(1):7-18.

[22] Brousse C., Boisaubert B. Quality of life and scales measuring. *Rev Med Int.,* 2007,28:58-462.

[23] Coons S. J., Rao S., Keininger D. L., et al. A comparative review of generic quality of life instruments. *Pharmacoeconomics*, 2000, 17:13-35.

[24] Guyatt G. H., Feeny D. H., Patrick D. L. Measuring health-related quality of life. *Ann Intern Med.*, 1993, 118:622-629.

[25] Seidl E. M. F., Zannon C. M. L. C. Qualidade de vida e saúde: aspectos conceituais e metodológicos. *Cad Saúde Públ.*, 2004, 20(2):580-588.

[26] Kluthcovsky A. C. G. C., Takayanagui A. M. M. Qualidade de vida – aspectos conceituais. *Rev Salus,* 2007, 1(1):13-15.

[27] Eustatia-Rutten C. F. A., et al. Quality of life in longterm exogenous subclinical hyperthyroidism and the effects of restoration of euthyroidism, a randomized controlled trial. *Clin Endocrinol.,* 2006, 64:284–291.

[28] Razvi S., McMillan C. V., Weaver J. U. Instruments used in measuring symptoms, health status and quality of life in hypothyroidism: a systematic qualitative review. *Clin Endocrinol.*, 2005, 63:617–624.

[29] Watt T., et al. Quality of life in patients with benign thyroid disorders - a review. *Eur J Endocrinol.*, 2006, 501–510.

[30] Donangelo I., Braunstein G. D. Update on Subclinical Hyperthyroidism. *Am Fam Physician,* 2011, 83(8):933-938.

[31] Teixeira P. F. S., et al. Avaliação clínica e de sintomas psiquiátricos no hipotireoidismo subclínico. *Rev Assoc Med Bras.*, 2006, 52(4):222-8.

[32] Cole D. P., Thase M. E., Mallinger A. G., et al. Slower Treatment Response in Bipolar Depression Predicted by Lower Pretreatment Thyroid Function. *Am J Psychiatry.,* 2002, 159:116-121.

[33] Teng C. T., Humes E. C., Demetrio F. N. Depressão e comorbidades clínicas. *Rev Psiqu Clin.*, 2005, 32(3):149-159.

[34] Nogueira C. R., Kimura E. T., et al. Hipotireoidismo: tratamento. *Diretrizes clínicas da Sociedade Brasileira de Endocrinologia e Metabolismo*. 2009,75-87.

[35] Mcmillan C., Bradley C., et al. Evaluation of new measures of the impact of hypothyroidism on quality of life and symptoms: the thydQoL and thySRQ. *Value Health.,* 2008, 11(2):285-294.

[36] Neves C., Alves M., et al. Doença de Graves. *Arquimed. Rev.,* 2008, 22(4/5):137-146.

[37] Grazia Y., Bülow A. R. Estudo da procedência dos pacientes e dos tipos de tireoidopatias encontradas no ambulatório de Endocrinologia do HSL-PUCRS nos anos de 2005 e 2006. *Scientia Medica*, 2006, 16(3):97-102.

[38] Acharya S. H. et al. Radioiodine therapy (RAI) for Graves' disease (GD) and the effect on ophthalmopathy: a systematic review. *Clin Endocrinol.,* 2008, 943-950.

[39] Scott I. U. et al. Functional status and quality of life measurement among ophthalmic patients. *Arch Ophthalmol.*, 1994, 112(3):329-335.

[40] Estcourt S. et al. The impact of thyroid eye disease upon patients' wellbeing: a qualitative analysis. *Clin Endocrinol.*, 2008, 68(4):635–639.

[41] Margolis M. K., et al.Vision specific instruments for the assessment of health-related quality of life and visual functioning - a literature review. *Pharmacoeconomics*, 2002, 20(12): 791-812.

[42] Gerding M. N., et al. Quality of life in patients with Graves' ophthalmopathy is markedly decreased: measurement by the medical outcomes study instrument. *Thyroid*, 1997, 7(6):885-889.

[43] Terwee C., et al. Long-term effects of Graves' ophthalmopathy on health-related quality of life. *Eur J Endocrinol.*, 2002, 146(6):751-757.

[44] Egle U. T., et al. The relevance of physical and psychosocial factors for the quality of life in patients with thyroid-associated orbitopathy (TAO). *Exp Clin Endocrinol Diabetes,* 1999, 107(5):168-171.

[45] Werner S. C. Modification of the classification of the eye changes of Graves' disease: recommendations of the Ad Hoc Committee of the American Thyroid Association. *J Clin Endocrinol Metab.*, 1977, 44(1):203-204.

[46] Wilson I. B., Cleary P. D. Linking clinical variables with health-related quality of life. A conceptual model of patient outcomes. *JAMA.,* 1995, 273(1):59-65.

[47] Magalhães C. H. T., Pereira M. D. et al. Auto-estima na forma inativa da oftalmopatia de Graves. *Arq Bras Oftalmol.*, 2008, 71(2):215-220.

[48] Andrade V. A., Gross J. L., et al. Tratamento do hipertireoidismo da doença de Graves. *Arq Bras Endocrinol Metab.*, 2001, 45(6):609-618.

[49] Terwee C. B., et al. Development of a disease specific quality of life questionnaire for patients with Graves' ophthalmopathy: the GO-QOL. *Brit J Ophthalmol.,* 1998, 773-779.

[50] Terwee C. B., et al. Interpretation and validity of changes in scores on the Graves' ophthalmology quality of life questionnaire (GO-QOL) after different treatments. *Clin Endocrinol.*, 2001, 391-398.

[51] Park J. J., et al. Assessing quality of life in Australian patients with Graves' ophthalmopathy. *Br J Ophthalmol.*, 2004, 88:75-78.

In: Quality of Life in Endocrine Diseases ISBN: 978-1-63463-911-8
Editor: Erika Cesar de Oliveira Naliato © 2015 Nova Science Publishers, Inc.

Chapter 8

Diabetes Mellitus and Quality of Life

Antonio C. M. Costa Jr. and Erika C. O. Naliato*

Center of Studies Ricardo A. T. Castilho of the Teresópolis Medical Association, Brazil

Abbreviations

ADA	American Diabetes Association
ARDS	Acute respiratory distress syndrome
BMI	Body mass index
CSII	Continuous subcutaneous insulin infusion
DM	Diabetes Mellitus
DMT1	Diabetes Mellitus type 1
DMT2	Diabetes Mellitus type 2
GI	Glucose intolerance
HRQL	Health-related quality of life
HbA1c	Glycated hemoglobin
IFG	Increased fasting glycemia
OGTT	Oral glucose tolerance test
LDL	Low density lipoprotein cholesterol
MCS	Mental Composite Scores

* Correspondence to: erikanaliato@uol.com.br.

MDI	Multiple daily injections
PedsQL	Pediatric Quality of Life Inventory
PCS	Physical Composite Scores and the mental evaluation
QoL	Quality of life
WHO	World Health Organization

Definition

As a group of metabolic disorders, the Diabetes Mellitus (DM) is basically characterized by chronic hyperglycemia associated with complications, dysfunctions and insufficiency of multiple systems of the body, where we can find disturbances on the metabolism of carbohydrates, fat, and proteins resulted from the malfunction in the secretion or action of insulin, or both [1].

Etiology

Despite the many different types of DM being characterized due to their etiology or specific pathogenesis, the cause of the most common types are still not completely acknowledged by the medical community. Most cases of DM are classified in two etiopathogenic categories (currently known as diabetes type 1 and diabetes type 2) [2, 3].

Etiological Types

The etiological classification of DM currently recommended by the World Health Organization (WHO) and by the American Diabetes Association (ADA) divides the disorder into four different groups: diabetes mellitus type 1 (DMT1), diabetes mellitus type 2 (DMT2), gestational diabetes, and other specific types (Table 1). This classification differs substantially from the previously used, which applied the terms *insulin-dependent* and *non-insulin-dependent*, no longer in use [4].

Diabetes Mellitus Type 1

It is the type of the disorder that primarily happens due to the destruction of the pancreatic beta cells, characterized for the total absence of insulin, normally autoimmune [3, 5].

Diabetes Mellitus Type 2

It is the most common type of DM in our society, characterized by the disorders of action and secretion of insulin (resistance and relative deficiency of insulin). However, even though the specific etiology is unknown, we recognized that there is no destruction of the pancreatic beta cells [1].

Gestational Diabetes

It is considered as the intolerance to carbohydrates associated to hyperglycemia with varying severity which begins or has its first appearance during pregnancy [3, 5]. This condition totally disappears after the birth of the child or the pregnancy interruption, and also is a risk factor to the development of DMT2.

Other Specific Types of Diabetes

Those in which the defect or the underlying disease process can be identified in a relatively specific way or those presenting other distinguished features. This category covers a variety of types of diabetes that are secondary to other specific conditions or associated with specific diseases or syndromes with distinct etiology [1].

Epidemiology

It is known that the epidemiological concepts include the prevalence rate (number of people with DM in a determined place, in a determined period), incidence rate (number of cases of diabetes in a place divided by a year), specific rate (when the incidence rate is calculated according to a specific characteristic such as age, gender, or race), and cumulative incidence (calculated from the specific incidence rate by age using life table methods) [1]. Regarding the difference of the epidemiological distribution of DM type 1 and type 2, the study of etiological factors considers the incidence rate the most informative measure for the frequency of diabetes in a population. The calculation of the incidence rate depends on the recognition and counting of new cases of diabetes: DMT1 can be easily identified, and virtually all the new cases are accounted for in the societies where people have access to medical assistance services. Conversely, the recognition of new cases of DMT2 depends on the seriousness of symptoms, the diagnosis activity of the health system, and the choice of the diagnosis criteria [6].

Table 1. Etiological classification of glycemia disturbs

Type 1 - destruction of beta-cells, usually leading to absolute insulin deficiency A - Auto-immune B – Idiopathic
Type 2 - may vary from insulin resistance to a secretory defect with or without insulin resistance
Other specific types Genetic defects of the beta-cell function Genetic defects in the insulin action Diseases of the exocrine pancreas Endocrinopathies Chemicals or drugs induced Infections Uncommon forms of immune-mediated diabetes Other genetic syndromes sometimes associated with diabetes
Gestational diabetes

Table 2. Specific Incidence rate by age of DM1 and DM2 for 100.000 people/year in Rochester (1960-69)

Age (in years)	Type 1	Type 2
0-09	6.5	0.0
10-19	12.5	7.5
20-29	9.5	9.5
30-39	6,9	66.8
40-49	17.3	155.4
50-59	25.8	322.2
60-69	26.9	612.8

Adapted from Kahn CR et al. (2009).

Data raised by medical assistance institutions in some cities in the USA show how the incidence rate of DMT 1 varies according to the age considering that the risk increases in the two decades of life, levels up in the third and fourth, and increases from then on, which demonstrates that there are two peaks of occurrence of DMT1. Conversely, the incidence rate of DMT2 increases steadily according to age, with elevations of almost 100 times, from childhood to old age, as it can be seen on table 2 [6].

Classification

Independently of etiology, DM goes through different clinical stages in its natural history which permits the identification of the disease even in those patients where etiology is unknown. When expressed in its completeness, DM is characterized by fasting hyperglycemia. Despite that, the disease may be recognized at other clinical stages through the glucose intolerance, as usually happens. In a long run, the effects of DM include lesion, dysfunction, and insufficiency of various organs (especially eyes, kidneys, heart, and blood vessels) [3].

The clinical classification presently adopted by the American Diabetes Association (ADA) and the World Health Organization (WHO) categorizes DM according to both clinical stages and etiological types (table 3).

The clinical stages reflect the notions that DM progresses through many stages during its natural history and individuals may move from one stage to another in any direction [3].

Table 3. Classification of DM according to the ADA and the WHO

Stages / Types	NORMOGLYCEMIA	HYPERGLYCEMIA			
	Normal tolerance to glucose	Glucose intolerance - GI or IFG	Diabetes Mellitus		
			Does not require insulin	Insulin for control	Insulin for survival
Diabetes Type 1	◄━━━━	━━━━	━━━━	━━━━	━━━━►
Diabetes Type 2*	◄────	────	────	────► ◄──	────►
Other specific types*	◄━━━━	━━━━	━━━━	━━━━►────	────►
Gestational Diabetes*	◄━━━━	━━━━	━━━━	━━━━►────	────►

*In rare cases, the patients may need insulin for survival.

Clinical Stages

Individuals who present diabetes go through various clinical stages during the development of the disease. Initially, the glucose regulation is normal and no glycemic abnormality can be identified, even if these individuals are submitted to an oral glucose tolerance test (OGTT). This stage is followed by a period of variable length where the glucose regulation is compromised. Patients who present some abnormality of the fasting glucose concentration, when receiving an OGTT may demonstrate glucose intolerance. Diabetes in itself is characterized by altered fasting glycemia or marking abnormalities in the glucose toleration, or both [3, 5].

Once diabetes is developed, the glycemia can be controlled in some patients, through changes in the lifestyle such as diet and increasing in physical activity, while in others, insulin or oral hypoglycemic agents are necessary to control or prevent ketosis and diabetic ketoacidosis (important emergency complications of the disease) [3, 5].

In all the kinds of diabetes, it is possible to have remission in the extension of hyperglycemia, especially if the diabetes is recent. This is observed more frequently in patients with DMT2 of recent start, for whom the intervention in lifestyle and/or aggressive initial glycemia treatment may result in visible reversion of abnormality with inversion of the glucose intolerance or its normalization [3, 5].

It is also possible to observe this phenomenon in patients with DMT1. The so-called 'honeymoon' period is identified when, after a short period of insulin treatment, there may be a variable period when insulin is no longer required for survival and tolerance to glucose may improve but, in the future, these patients will need insulin for survival [3, 5].

The regulation of the compromised glucose refers to the intermediate metabolic stage between normal glucose homeostasis and diabetes, which may be identified by glucose intolerance (GI) or increased fasting glycemia (IFG) [3, 5].

Some care must be taken in relation to that since GI and IFG are not synonyms and may represent different abnormalities of the glucose regulation, although they may occur at the same time. For instance, individuals with any of these compromised states of glucose regulation have a risk to diabetes progression [10, 11], considering that the GI confirmation can only be made with TOTG, and IFG refers to the concentrations of fasting glucose that are lower than those necessary for the diagnosis of diabetes, although higher than those generally found in people with normal glucose tolerance. People with GI or AFG have normal levels or slight elevated rises of glycated hemoglobin [12], where GI is frequently associated with the presence of other indicators of the metabolic syndrome or insulin resistance [13].

Symptomatology

The patient with DM may present characteristic symptoms such as thirst, polyuria, bleary eyesight, somnolence or coma, inexplicable weight loss, accentuated glycosuria, and polyphagia. In its most serious forms, we may encounter the patient with diabetic ketoacidosis or nonketotic hyperosmolarity which if not effectively treated, may lead to stupor, coma, and death. Frequently, the symptoms do not manifest themselves in a serious fashion and may even be absent [1, 3, 5].

Diagnosis

The diagnosis is normally done in routine blood or urine test, or in the manifestation of a complication (since the symptoms are not always present and hyperglycemia may be evident for insufficient time to generate complications, before the diagnosis is reached) [1, 3, 5].

Despite that, the diagnosis criteria established by ADA include: glycemia (randomly collected) higher or equal to 200mg/dl, associated with signals/symptoms compatible with DM, fasting glycemia equal or higher to 126mg/dl in more than one occasion and/or OGTT with glycemia evaluation 2h after 75g of glucose by mouth equal or higher to 200mg/dl on more than one occasion [1, 3, 5].

Treatment

The treatment of DMT1 involves the exogenous replacement of insulin where three different treatment schemes may be used: two daily applications (2/3 of daily dose of NPH insulin in the morning injection and 1/3 in nocturnal injection), multiple daily applications (40-50% of the dose administered as NPH insulin or long duration analogues in the morning and before sleep or as glargine insulin in one single daily dose, and the remaining 50-60% divided in three doses that must be administered with regular or ultrafast insulin), and the continuous infusion of insulin (under the form of regular or, preferably, ultrafast insulin) [1].

The treatment of DMT2 includes the use of oral antidiabetic drugs with or without exogenous insulin replacement. They aim for the glycemic control seeking the reduction to values close to the glycemia normal zone (pre-prandial: 80-120 mg/dl, when going to bed: 100-140 mg/dl, glycosylated hemoglobin (HbA1c): lower than 7%) [1].

Complications

The complications of DM may be the result of the disease itself and /or the treatment adopted by the patient. The complications of the disease are divided in macrovascular (cardiac, cerebrovascular, and peripheral arterial diseases), and microvascular as retinopathy, nephropathy, neuropathy, and diabetic gangrene (diabetic foot gangrene) [1, 3, 5].

The complications related to the treatment or the absence, or inadequacy of it include hypoglycemia, diabetic ketoacidosis, cerebral edema, hyperchloremic metabolic acidosis, hyperosmolar nonketotic state, and acute respiratory distress syndrome (ARDS - inflammatory syndrome of the alveolar-capillary membrane, of sudden start, with the increase of capillary permeability, characterized by hypoxemia, the presence of bilateral pulmonary infiltrates in chest X-ray, and absence of clinical findings of left cardiac failure) [1 ,3, 5].

Quality of Life in the Patient with Diabetes Mellitus

'Quality of life' (QoL - quality of life) is a concept that gathers an ample range of experiences of the human being. On the medical aspect, it is related to the effects of a disease on a patient, being the health-related quality of life (HRQL) the focus of studies that evaluate the quality of life of patients with specific diseases [14].

For a long time, DM has been considered a biopsychosocial disease and is, nowadays, one of the most important chronic diseases in the world population. It is related to vascular complications with elevated morbidity and mortality.

In this case, it is a world consensus that the ideal treatment for the disease must prevent the chronic complications while preserving a good QoL of the patient [14].

The treatment of the disease involves a brutal change in the patient's lifestyle, including the maintenance of a low level of blood glucose with a low-carb level diet, regular physical activity, daily monitoring of glycemia by glucometers, regular laboratory tests, and constant administration of oral drugs or insulin supplements [14].

In a study with 400 diabetic patients, the authors evaluated demographic status in relation to the patients' general health, their mental health and behaviour, beliefs, knowledge, and satisfaction in relation to the treatment of DM. Patients who reported difficulty of access to basic attention, DM complications, comorbidities associated with the disease, and dissatisfaction with health service presented a worse health related quality of life (HRQL). Conversely, those patients with difficulty of access to basic attention, high levels of cholesterol, and comorbidities associated with the disease, presented a better HRQL on the hypothetic absence of the disease [14].

Factors That Influence the Quality of Life of Patients with Diabetes Mellitus

The study of Luzny & Ivanova (2009) shows us that right after the Second World War, the material and economic conditions represented great influence on the perception of the QoL of an individual. At that time, having a job and good life conditions were pre-requisites for a good QoL. Later, with the greater development of medicine and society, new factors that influenced QoL have been taken into consideration, such as social, political, psychological, environmental, and spiritual aspects associated with the demands of lifestyle.

Table 4. Factors that influence quality of life

Health and health-related Aspects
Material and Economic Aspects
Psychological Aspects
Spiritual Aspects
Social Aspects and Social Networks
Environmental Aspects
Political Aspects
New Lifestyle

DM has been associated with a low QoL that tends to decrease more and more over the years [15, 16]. Many studies have identified clinical and demographic characteristics, disease representations, and behaviours that interfere with the health associated with the HRQL in patients with diabetes. Many characteristics were associated with low HRQL in patients with diabetes, including the low socioeconomic status, medical comorbidities, complications and symptoms related to DM, the higher value of body mass index (BMI), pain, depression, anxiety, lower perception of the DM control, low self-efficiency, pessimism, non-commitment to a diet that includes physical activity, and a continuity of the assistance that may be considered bad [16-27].

Many studies demonstrate that the QoL of patients with DM decreases over their lives and the presence of complications and comorbidities of the disease have an additional negative impact in the QoL of these patients [28].

The study of Costa Jr et al. (2011) compared the difference in QoL of diabetic and non-diabetic patients hospitalized in Brazil, finding lower physical capacity, reduction in the general health, and low social functioning scores in diabetic patients. Besides that, the patients with diabetes presented a high prevalence of hypertension and ischemic heart disease [28].

In this study, the patients with diagnosis of hypertension also presented a decrease in the scores related to physical capacity, general health, and social functioning; despite that, the patients with ischaemic heart disease were the ones that presented the worst scores of the categories mentioned above. Nevertheless, a multivariate analysis demonstrated that hypertension was considered the disease with the highest influence in the physical capacity of diabetic patients, while ischaemic heart disease influenced in the general health and the social functioning of these patients [28]. This study confirms previous researches and of higher dimension conducted in different populations of diabetics, where the cardiovascular complications and comorbidities were pointed out as the main determiners in the reduction of HRQL in diabetic patients [28].

Quality of Life in Children and Adolescents with Diabetes Mellitus

Due to the high prevalence of young people (children and adolescents) presenting diabetes mellitus, many studies were developed to analyse the QoL in this group of patients, including Naughton's et al. (2008) that shows some considerably relevant data.

Young patients with DM find unique difficulties in their lives, considering that besides all the stressful factors that we usually deal with during this stage of life, young people with DM find problems and physical and social limitations associated to the disease [29-35]. In addition, conflicts deriving from the treatment generate more stress between parents and their children which may aggravate the patient's condition [36, 37].

Children and adolescents who show a better adjustment to DM right after the diagnoses were associated with better long term-results [38, 39]. The youngest patients were also associated with better self-control of the glucose and QoL levels [40, 41]. Despite that, during adolescence, social competitions, school, and other demands affect negatively the commitment to the treatment [29, 42-44].

Many studies suggest that girls have worse metabolic control than boys due to the low adherence to treatment [29, 45]. Other works demonstrated that adolescents with worse metabolic control present a higher occurrence of psychopathy [46-48] and consequent reduction in the QoL [29, 39, 49].

Naughton et al. (2008) analyzed the pediatric QoL with the PedsQL (*Pediatric Quality of Life Inventory*). They found a significantly higher (better) result in young people with DMT1 when compared to young people with DMT2 in all items and sub-items evaluated. In the group with DMT1, the score analysis by PedsQL detected a difference in the QoL in relation to gender and age, where the older groups demonstrated a low QoL in the feminine gender and a high QoL in the masculine. A better result on the PedsQL was found in groups that used an insulin pump when compared to groups that injected subcutaneous insulin bolus in the traditional manner. Users of the insulin pump had a level of HbA1c inferior to 9%, did not present comorbidities, and possessed one or fewer hospital or emergency confinements over the last 6 months. Race/ethnicity, parents' education, DM length, and BMI were the aspects evaluated in this study which did not show significant different results concerning global HRQL of this group.

Conversely, in the group with DMT2, few co-variables were significantly associated with the QoL. When compared with the use of oral medications for diabetes, the injection of insulin at least three times/day was significantly associated with a better HRQL. Meanwhile, two or more visits to the emergency room over the last six months were significantly associated with a worse HRQL. The demographic variables, DM length, level of HbA1c, BMI, complications, and comorbidities were not significantly associated with the QoL of this group.

Naughton et al. (2008) mentioned that concerning gender, a longer duration of the disease was associated with a better global HRQL in the masculine group, while two or more visits to the emergency room (as a result of emergencies) compared to none were associated with a worse HRQL in the feminine group.

It is possible to state that the main finding of this study was the young people with DMT2 presenting a HRQL significantly lower than the ones with DMT1. In the group of patients with DMT2, the use of injectable insulin was also associated with better emotional, educational, and psychosocial functionalities, suggesting the existence of an important psychosocial component of the treatment adopted by the patients. It is plausible that the young people of this group that used oral medications and/or established changes in diet and treatment experienced a glycemic control inferior to the ideal, which may affect their psychosocial and physical functionalities, as observed in previous studies developed with children with DMT1 [30, 36, 40, 50]. A better flexibility in relation to treatment of diabetes in schools may be of great importance [51]. Between the young people with DMT1, a better global HRQL was more strongly associated with the fact of having a private health plan, better glycemic control, and less comorbidities, as concluded in previous studies [40, 38, 49, 52-55].

The interaction between gender and age found by Naughton et al. (2008) indicated that young people of the feminine gender have a worse HRQL on the older groups while the older young people of the masculine gender presented a better HRQL, which is also in accordance with the previous studies [49, 52]. Therefore, it can be concluded that, as approaching puberty and adolescence, the girls tend to experience stronger social and personal pressure, which may affect their QoL and the maintenance of the DM.

The results of the study suggest that doctors must be alert to the potential detriment of the QoL of young people after the diagnosis of DMT1 or DMT2, particularly between the girls. The patients' age, their social environment and financial resources, the kind of treatment, and the severity of the condition of each one affects the daily maintenance of the diabetes. As a result, developing in the clinical practice some form of support that helps young people to deal better with the DM and increases their cooperation with the treatment has the potential of establishing a better HRQL in pediatric patients [56].

Quality of Life in Elderly People Carriers of Diabetes Mellitus

Diabetes Mellitus is a disease with high prevalence also in the elderly population. The number of diabetic elderly patients should double over the next 20-30 years. Only in the United Kingdom, for instance, the elderly population represents more than half of the individuals with DM [57]. Besides, the increase in life expectancy means a higher decrease in the QoL due to complications. Older people with diabetes end up experiencing substantial comorbidities [57, 58], physical incapacitation [59], and psychological disorders, which include impaired cognitive function [57, 60], low social independence [57], and a rise in the use of the health services [61].

Trief et al. (2003) developed a study using the SF-36 questionnaire as a research tool in order to compare the HRQL between elderly patients and younger adults with DMT2. There was not much difference in the evaluation of the physical and mental scores; nevertheless, elderly patients showed a larger limitation due to physical problems and yet, revealed a better social function. In the diabetes-specific evaluation, the older ones demonstrated more satisfaction with aspects of their lives related to the disease. In addition, they demonstrated lower emotional anguish and better ability to deal with the disease.

In this study, the physical evaluation (*PCS – Physical Composite Scores*) and the mental evaluation (*MCS – Mental Composite Scores*) were analysed and calculated through SF-36. The PCS evaluates the general physical health state of the patient while the MCS evaluates the patient's general mental health state [62]. In this analysis, the patients were divided into two groups: patients aged between 30 and 65 and patients aged 65 or above. In the PCS analysis, adults obtained a higher result (better HRQL) than the elderly ones, representing the limitations the older ones have due to physical problems. Despite that, in the analysis of the MCS results, the elderly obtained a result superior to the non-elderly adults, which demonstrates a better social function.

Since the type of diabetes is associated with age, and the latter influences some aspects of HRQL, it is possible that this type may also predict the QoL. It was considering this that Trief et al. (2003) decided to analyse the QoL according to the type of DM of their research subjects. The results demonstrated that the carriers of DMT2 presented a physical functionality significantly worse than the DMT1 patients, as well as a lower vitality and higher quantities of limitations in consequence of emotional problems. Despite that, they demonstrated a better social functionality. Also, the interaction coefficient between age and type of DM was tested for each value found but no significant statistical interactions were found, which implies that age does not depend on the type of diabetes in order to predict HRQL.

Many times, we assume that getting old is linked to more anguish and pessimism due to physical, emotional, and social losses - a hypothesis supported by classical well-being researches [63, 64]. However, recent works established that older people are not unhappy [69, 70], and well-being seems to improve with age [67-69], generating the hypothesis that older adults manage to regulate their emotions more efficiently and conduct their lives in order to minimize negative emotions while maximizing the positive ones [69]. This aspect helps to explain the results of Trief et al. (2003), where the differences that appeared in the comparison between the group of adults and the group of elderly people suggest that despite experimenting more restrictions, the elderly people carriers of DM feel they can deal with such limitations and, therefore, manage the anguishes and demands of the diabetes lifestyle [70].

Influence of Treatment in the Quality of Life of the Patient with Diabetes Mellitus

Concerning the treatment, two studies compared the effects on QoL according to the patient's treatment. In the first one, with the analysis of drug treatment with oral antidiabetics combined or not with insulin, a result of worse HRQL was found when compared to pure dietary treatment. In the second study, a gradational damage in QoL was also found, despite the treatment adopted (diet, pills, and/or insulin); however, this association disappeared when it was adjusted to other evaluation factors, which did not happen in the first study [71-73].

In a study conducted in Nordic countries, it was concluded that DM exerts a great negative impact in the QoL of men and women, mostly due to the necessity of eating habits alterations, once the patients claim they do not appreciate the food and do not have freedom to eat and drink [74].

Influence of Glycemic Control in the Quality of Life

Nicolucci et al. (2008) compared QoL and the satisfaction in relation to treatment in adults with DMT1 treated with continuous subcutaneous insulin infusion (CSII) versus multiple daily injections (MDI). This work demonstrated that despite having more severe diseases (high prevalence of complications and longer diabetes duration), patients treated with CSII had HbA1c levels almost identical to those individuals treated with MDI, with no negative impact in the QoL. Besides, patients treated with CSII showed a lower perception to diabetes-specific restrictions and responsibilities. These findings are similar to a previous randomized study that compares CSII vs. MDI NPH-exclusive, showing that patients treated with CSII felt less restrained on the aspects related to diet and daily activities [75].

The diabetes and its treatments affect negatively the patient's QoL, particularly in relation to the dietary restriction imposed by the traditional treatment regime [76]. Effective treatment strategies must allow patients to reach a good glycemic control without significantly interfering with the independence and flexibility of each one's lifestyle. The ability to increase the treatment's flexibility in order to follow up the patient's different moments of the day is the most frequent reason cited by individuals who chose CSII [77], as it allows the patient to modify the available insulin in a matter of minutes, which permits the execution of activities that would be risky otherwise, such as missing or delaying of meals, sleeping late in weekends, or even the practice of heavy physical exercises. Besides, the study revealed that the use of CSII was also associated to a significantly higher score in relation to satisfaction with the treatment comparing with individuals treated both with the MDI glargine-exclusive or the MDI NPH-exclusive regimes.

In studies that evaluated the satisfaction with the treatment with the use of different research instruments, multiple results were found. In particular, the treatment with CSII was associated with better satisfaction scores in one study [75], while in other, few differences were found [78]. Without a doubt, hypoglycemia is a constant worry of diabetic patients and the fear of hypoglycemia episodes may affect negatively the acceptance of insulin therapy and the capacity of reduction of the HbA1c levels over an intensive treatment [79]. One important observation in the study mentioned above is the verification of a reduction in the fear of hypoglycemia episodes on patients treated with CSII. This fact corresponds to the findings of a previous study which demonstrates that the switch to the CSII treatment over the MDI NPH-exclusive was associated to a reduction in the incidence of hypoglycemia episodes and a parallel reduction of the fear of hypoglycemia episodes [80].

As a result, this study confirmed the findings of previous smaller scope researches which have suggested that CSII is not associated with the deterioration of the QoL. On the contrary, in both genders, it is associated with a lower perception of the disease as a burden and with a high satisfaction with the treatment when compared with the MDI NPH-exclusive. In addition, this is the first ample spectrum study suggesting an improvement in the QoL due to the great flexibility on the lifestyle, less fear of hypoglycemia, and higher satisfaction in the treatment when CSII is compared with the MDI glargine-exclusive regime [81].

Quality of Life and Adherence to the Treatment of Diabetes

In 2001, the World Health Organization prepared a meeting in order to approach the 'adherence to therapy' problem. The definition of 'adherence to long-term therapy' adopted was: point in which the individual behaviour of making use of medications, following a diet and/or making changes in the lifestyle corresponds to the recommendation proposed by the health professionals [82]. We know that to obtain a satisfactory adherence to the treatment patients must have an adequate knowledge about self-care [83], and that each one's attitudes have an important role in this process of change which generates adherence to therapy, since they predict and explain the human behaviour [84].

When the diabetics do not adhere to their prescriptions, the efficiency of the medications decreases [85] as well as their glycemic control. When this occurs, there is a higher risk of manifestations of chronic and/or acute complications [86, 87] leading to unnecessary hospital admissions [88]. A systematic review about the adherence to drug treatment of diabetes presented frequencies from 36% to 93% [89]. In addition, while some studies show a relation between the QoL and the glycemic control [90-92], other researches demonstrate that no such connection exists [93-96]. Therefore, the hypothesis that adherence to drug treatment and QoL are interconnected was suggested, although some contradictory results appear in different works [97-101].

A research developed by Martínez et al. (2008) evaluated the association between the QoL and the patients' behaviour in relation to the adherence to treatment, the knowledge of medical prescriptions, attitude towards adherence to therapy, and the combination of knowledge and attitude in patients with DMT2. There were no remarkable differences in the general analysis of the six domains of the QoL with the behaviour of patients related to the adherence to treatment. Despite that, when combined, the strong knowledge about the subject (disease and prescription) and the positive attitude towards the treatment generate an important difference in the general results of five out of the six areas (physical, psychological, level of independence, social relation, and environment). Differently from a study with the Mexican population which demonstrated a 50% adherence on patients with DMT2 [102, 103], only 17.2% of the patients of Martínez et al. (2008) demonstrated a good behaviour related to the adherence to therapy. Therefore, we may consider important the exploration of the psychological precursors of the individual behaviour in the adherence to therapy, since the knowledge and comprehension of the prescriptions and the disease along with the patients' positivity on thoughts and attitudes interfere productively in their QoL [104].

Relation between Life Expectancy, Mortality and Quality of Life

Brown et al. (2008) affirm that the present criteria for DM recommend that patients keep the glycosylated hemoglobin (HbA1c) inferior to 7% [105], blood pressure inferior or equal to 130/80 mmHg [106], and LDL cholesterol (low density lipoprotein cholesterol) below 100 mg/dL [107] to minimize the risk of development of micro- and macrovascular complications [108-110]. However, the reach of these levels and the minimization of these risk factors require a number of medications that may increase progressively according to the duration of the patient's disease [111, 112].

Some studies have already investigated the relation between HRQL and the mortality of diabetic patients. Despite that, they have always presented some point of disagreement. The recent research of Landman et al. (2010) revised this association but with a longer follow-up period than the others (around 10 years), with a special focus on the elderly population (aged above 75) and the possible differences between the genders [114].

The research tool used was the RAND-36, considered a generic research instrument since it evaluates the health aspects relevant to any functional and social states of an individual [62, 113]. The RAND-36 nine scores can be divided into two already known evaluations: physical evaluation (*PCS – Physical Composite Scores*) and mental evaluation (*MCS – Mental Composite Scores*) [62]. A low score in PCS indicates a substantial limitation in the self-care, physical and social activities, considerable corporal pain, or frequent fatigue. In MCS, a low score indicates frequent psychological anguish and considerable limitation on the role of the social function due to emotional problems [114].

The results of Landman et al. (2010) demonstrate that, after an approximately 10-year follow-up period, the total and cardiovascular mortality increased for patients with DMT2 that presented a HRQL on the base line. Both PCS and MCS were related with the total and cardiovascular mortality despite the differences in gender and age. According to the authors' analysis, it did not become evident whether there is a true relation between HRQL and mortality, since a reduction in the HRQL was associated with the increase of the mortality (total or cardiovascular) between adult and elderly patients with DMT2. The question that remains is whether the HRQL is a modifiable risk factor or just a burden of the disease. Therefore, the instruments that evaluate the HRQL may become a tool of extreme clinical utility, not only to identify patients with low HRQL, but also to indicate those that present an elevation in the mortality risk [114].

Conclusion

The QoL of a human being is such an ample concept that involves a range of diverse experiences. In medicine, it is related to the effects of a disease on a patient, being the health related QoL (HRQL) the focus of the majority of the studies in this area [10].

Diabetes Mellitus is considered a biopsychosocial disease and is one of the most important chronic infirmities in the world population at the moment. It is related to micro- and macrovascular alterations and/or complications that increase substantially both morbidity and mortality and usually tend to generate a considerable drop in their QoL [10]. When study groups are differentiated according to age, we clearly observe that the adult population (especially the elderly) has a considerably bigger psychological support when compared to the young people [69]. And, together with all the stressful factors usually found in adolescence, young people with DM present both physical as well as social problems and limitations associated with the disease. It is observed that those with DMT2 present a significantly lower HRQL than the ones with DMT1 and, when approaching puberty and adolescence, girls tend to experience higher social and personal pressure than boys, which affects both their QoL as well as the DM maintenance [56].

As a result, the treatment of the disease, which must be specific to each individual and generally involves a great change in the patient's lifestyle (including various changes in habits and behaviours many times created or acquired during a whole life), faces a serious obstacle: the adhesion to treatment which, if not adequately operated, many times makes the therapy ineffective [104].

Also, as mentioned by Landman et al. (2010): the question that remains is whether HRQL is a modifiable risk factor or just a burden of the Diabetes Mellitus [114].

References

[1] Kahn C. R. et al. Epidemiologia do diabetes mellitus: Warram JH, Krolewski AS (eds). *Joslin: Diabetes Mellitus*, 14th ed. Porto Alegre, Brazil: Artmed; 2009:355-358.

[2] Harris M. I. et al. Comparison of diabetes diagnostic categories in the U.S. population, according do 1997 American Diabetes Association and 1980-1985 World Health Organization diagnostic criteria. *Diabetes Care*, 1997, 20:1859-1862.

[3] Gavin J. R. et al. Report of the Expert Committee on the Diagnosis and Classification of Diabetes Mellitus. *Diabetes Care*, 1997, 20:1183-1197.

[4] WHO Study Group. Diabetes mellitus. *Technical Report Series 727*. Geneva: World Health Organization, 1985.

[5] WHO Consultation Group. Part 1: Diagnosis and classification of diabetes mellitus. *Definition, diagnosis and classification of diabetes mellitus and its complications*. 2nd edition. WHO/NCD/NCS. Geneva: World Health Organization; 1999:1-59.

[6] Rothman K. J. & Greenland S. Measures of disease frequency. Rothman K. J., Greenland S. (eds). *Modern epidemiology*. 2nd edition. Philadelphia, USA: Lippincott-Raven Publishers; 1998: 29-46.

[7] Savage P. J. et al. Normalization of insulin and glucagon secretion in ketosis-resistant diabetes mellitus with prolonged diet therapy. *J Clin Endocrinol Metab.*, 1979, 49:830-833.

[8] Agner T. et al. Remission in IDDM: prospective study of basal C-peptide and insulin dose in 268 consecutive patients. *Diabetes Care*, 1987, 10:164-169.

[9] O'Sullivan J. B. Diabetes mellitus after GDM. *Diabetes*, 1991, 40 [Suppl 2]:131-135, 1991.

[10] Gabir M. M. et al. The 1997 American Diabetes Association and 1999 World Health Organization criteria for hyperglycemia in the diagnosis and prediction of diabetes. *Diabetes Care*, 2002, 23:1108-1112.

[11] De Vegt F. et al. Relation of impaired fasting and post load glucose with incident type 2 diabetes in a Dutch population: The Hoorn Study. *JAMA*, 2001, 285: 2109-2113.

[12] Harris M. I. et al. Prevalence of diabetes, impaired fasting glucose, and impaired glucose tolerance in U.S. adults. The Third National Health and Nutrition Examination Survey; 1988-1994. *Diabetes Care*, 1998, 21:518-524.

[13] Defronzo R. A. & Ferrannini E. Insulin Resistance: a multifaceted syndrome responsible for NIDDM, obesity, hypertension, dyslipidemia and atherosclerotic cardiovascular disease. *Diabetes Care*, 1991, 14:173-194.

[14] DeCoster V. A. Challenges of type 2 diabetes and the role of health care social workers: A neglected area of practice. *Health & Social Work*, 2001, 26:26-37.

[15] Brown D. W. et al. Diabetes mellitus and health-related quality of life among older adults. Findings from the behavioral risk factor surveillance system (BRESS). *Diabetes Research and Clinical Practice*, 2004, 65:105-115.

[16] Hart H. E. et al. Factors that predicted change in health-related quality of life were identified in a cohort of diabetes mellitus type 1 patients. *J Clin Epidemiol.*, 2005, 58:1158—1164.

[17] Wandell P. E. Quality of life of patients with diabetes mellitus. An overview of research in primary health care in the Nordic countries. *Scand J Primary Health Care*, 2005, 23:68-74.

[18] Davis R. E. et al. Impact of hypoglycemia on quality of life and productivity in type 1 and type 2 diabetes. *Curr Med Res Opinion*, 2005, 27:1477-1483.

[19] De Berardis G. et al. Erectile dysfunction and quality of life in type 2 diabetic patients: A serious problem too often overlooked. *Diabetes Care*, 2002, 25:284-291.

[20] Vileikyte L. Diabetic foot ulcers: A quality of life issue. *Diabetes Metab Res Rev.*, 2001, 17:246-249.

[21] Maddigan S. L. et al. Understanding the complex associations between patient-provider relationships, self-care behaviors, and health-related quality of life in type 2 diabetes: A structural equation modeling approach. *Qual Life Res.*, 2005, 14:1489-1500.

[22] Lustman P. J. & Clouse R. E. Depression in diabetic patients: The relationship between mood and glycemic control. *J Diabetes Complications*, 2005, 19:113-122.

[23] Paschalides C. et al. The associations of anxiety, depression and personal illness representations with glycemic control and health-related quality of life in patients with type 2 diabetes mellitus. *J Psychosom Res.*, 2004, 51:557-564.

[24] Rose M. et al. The network of psychological variables in patients with diabetes and their importance for quality of life and metabolic control. *Diabetes Care*, 2002, 25:35-42.

[25] Glasgow R. Quality of life and associated characteristics in a large national sample of adults with diabetes. *Diabetes Care*, 1997, 20:562-567.

[26] Smith D. W. & McFall S. L. The relationship of diet and exercise for weight control and the quality of life gap associated with diabetes. *J Psychosom Res.*, 2005, 59:385-392.

[27] Luzny J. & Ivanova K. Quality of life in hospitalized seniors with psychiatric disorders (a cross-sectional study from the Kromeriz District, Czech Republic). *Biomed Pap Med Fac Univ Palacky Olomouc Czech Repub.*, 2009, 153(4):315–318.

[28] Costa Jr, A. C. M. et al. Diabetes and Quality of life in Hospitalized Patients. *Endocr Rev.*, 2011, 32 (03_MeetingAbstracts): P1-526.

[29] Cameron F. J. The impact of diabetes on health-related quality of life in children and adolescents. *Pediatr Diabetes*, 2003, 4(3):132-136.

[30] Hesketh K. D. et al. Health-related quality of life and metabolic control in children with type 1 diabetes: a prospective cohort study. *Diabetes Care*, 2004, 27(2):415-420.

[31] Huang G. H. et al. Wisconsin Diabetes Registry. Self-rated health among young people with type 1 diabetes in relation to risk factors in a longitudinal study. *Am J Epidemiol.*, 2004, 159(4):364-372.

[32] Sawyer S. M. et al. Adolescents with a chronic condition: challenges living, challenges treating. *Lancet*, 2007, 369(9571):1481-1489.

[33] Pinhas-Hamiel O. & Zeitler P. Acute and chronic complications of type 2 diabetes mellitus in children and adolescents. *Lancet*, 2007, 369(9575):1823-1831.

[34] De Wit M. et al. Self-report and parent-report of physical and psychosocial well-being in Dutch adolescents with type 1 diabetes in relation to glycemic control. *Health Qual Life Outcomes*, 2007, 5:10-18.

[35] Curtis J. A. & Hagerty D. Managing diabetes in childhood and adolescence. *Can Fam Physician*, 2002, 48:499-502 and 505-509.

[36] Laffel L. M. B. et al. General quality of life in youth with type 1 diabetes: relationship to patient management and diabetes-specific conflict. *Diabetes Care*, 2003, 26(11):3067-3073.

[37] Grey M. et al. Personal and family factors associated with quality of life in adolescents with diabetes. *Diabetes Care*, 1998, 21(6):909-914.

[38] Northam E. Psychosocial and family functioning in children with insulin-dependent diabetes at diagnosis and one year later. *J Pediatr Psychol.*, 1996, 21(5):699-717.

[39] Kovacs M. et al. Psychiatric disorder and metabolic control among youths with IDDM: a longitudinal study. *Diabetes Care*, 1996, 19(4):318-323.

[40] Wagner V. M. et al. Age, metabolic control and type of insulin regime influences health-related quality of life in children and adolescents with type 1 diabetes mellitus. *Eur J Pediatr.*, 2005, 164(8):491-496 2005.

[41] Anderson B et al. Parental involvement in diabetes management tasks: relationships to blood glucose monitoring adherence and metabolic control in young adolescents with insulin-dependent diabetes mellitus. *J Pediatr.*, 1997, 130(2):257-265.

[42] Du Pasquier-Fediaevsky L. & Tubiana-Rufi N. PEDIAB Collaborative Group. Discordance between physician and adolescent assessments of adherence to treatment: influence of HbA1c level. *Diabetes Care*, 1999, 22(9):1445-1449.

[43] Carroll A. E., Marrero D. G. The role of significant others in adolescent diabetes: a qualitative study. *Diabetes Educ.*, 2006, 32(2):243-252.

[44] Bryden K. S. et al. Clinical and psychological course of diabetes from adolescence to young adulthood. *Diabetes Care*, 2001, 24(9):1536-1540.

[45] Nurick M. A., Johnson S. B. Enhancing blood glucose awareness in adolescents and young adults with IDDM. *Diabetes Care*, 1991, 14(1):1-7.

[46] Blanz B. J. et al. IDDM is a risk factor for adolescent psychiatric disorders. *Diabetes Care*, 1993, 16(12):1579-1587.

[47] La Greca A. M. et al. Adolescents with diabetes: gender differences in psychological functioning and glycemic control. *Child Health Care*, 1995, 24(1):61-78.

[48] Hassan K. et al. The role of socioeconomic status, depression, quality of life, and glycemic control in type 1 diabetes mellitus. *J Pediatr.*, 2006, 149(4):526-531.

[49] Guttmann-Bauman I. et al. Metabolic control and quality-of-life self-assessment in adolescents with IDDM. *Diabetes Care*, 1998, 21(6):915-918.

[50] Wake M. et al. The Child Health Questionnaire in children with diabetes: cross-sectional survey of parent and adolescent-reported functional health status. *Diabet Med.*, 2000, 17(10).700-707.

[51] Wagner J. et al. Brief report: glycemic control, quality of life, and school experiences among students with diabetes. *J Pediatr Psychol.*, 2006, 31(8):764-769.

[52] Hoey H. et al. Good metabolic control is associated with better quality of life in 2101 adolescents with type 1 diabetes. *Diabetes Care*, 2001, 24(11):1923-1928.

[53] McMahon S. K. et al. Insulin pump therapy in children and adolescents: improvements in key parameters of diabetes management including quality of life. *Diabet Med.*, 2005, 22(1):92-96.

[54] Wagner V. M. et al. Age, metabolic control and type of insulin regime influences health-related quality of life in children and adolescents with type 1 diabetes mellitus. *Eur J Pediatr.*, 2005, 164(8):491-496.

[55] Arif A. A., Rohrer J. E. The relationship between obesity, hyperglycemia symptoms, and health-related quality of life among Hispanic and non-Hispanic white children and adolescents. *BMC Fam Pract.*, 2006, 7:3-10.

[56] Naughton M. J. et al. Health-Related Quality of Life of Children and Adolescents With Type 1 or Type 2 Diabetes Mellitus. SEARCH for Diabetes in Youth Study. *Arch Pediatr Adolesc Med.*, 2008, 162(7):649-657.

[57] Dornan T. L. et al. A community survey of diabetes in the elderly. *Diabetic Med.*, 1992, 9:860–865, 1992.

[58] Moritz D. J. et al. The health burden of diabetes for the elderly in four communities. *Public Health Rep.*, 1994, 109:782–790.

[59] Gregg E. W. et al. Diabetes and physical disability among older U.S. adults. *Diabetes Care*, 2000, 23:1272–1277.

[60] Reaven G. M. et al. Relationship between hyperglycemia and cognitive function in older NIDDM patients. *Diabetes Care*, 1990, 13:16–21.

[61] Pulsinelli W. A. et al. Increased damage after ischemic stroke in patients with and without established diabetes mellitus. *Am J Med.*, 1983, 74:540–544.

[62] Ware Jr J. E. et al. *SF-36 Physical and Mental Health Summary Scales: A User's Manual.* The Health Institute, New England Medical Center. Boston, USA: 1994.

[63] Andrews F. M., Withey S. B. *Social Indicators of Well-Being: America's Perception of Life Quality*. Plenum, New York, USA: 1976.

[64] Ryff C. D., Keyes C. L. M. The structure of psychological wellbeing revisited. *J Pers Soc Psychol.*, 1995, 69:719–727.

[65] Brandstadter J., Greve W. The aging self: Stabilizing and protective processes. *Dev Rev.*, 1994, 14:52–80.

[66] Filipp S. H. Motivation and emotion. Birren JE; Schaie KW (eds). *Handbook of the Psychology of Aging.* San Diego, USA: Academic Press; 1996:218–235.

[67] Carstensen L. L., Turk-Charles S. The salience of emotion across the adult life span. *Psychol Aging*, 1994, 9:259–64.

[68] Lawton M. P. Quality of life and affect in later life. Magai C; McFadden SH (eds). *Handbook of Emotion, Adult Development and Aging*. San Diego, USA: Academic Press; 1996:327–348.

[69] Mroczek D. K., Kolarz C. M. The effect of age on positive and negative affect: A developmental perspective on happiness. *J Pers Soc Psychol.*, 1998, 75:1333–1349.

[70] Trief P. M. et al. A comparison of health-related quality of elderly and younger insulin-treated adults with diabetes. *Age and Aging*, 2003, 32:613-618.

[71] Keinanen-Kiukaanniemi S. et al. Health related quality of life in diabetic patients measured by the Nottingham Health Profile. *Diabet Med.*, 1996, 13:382-388.

[72] Wandell P. E. et al. Quality of life among diabetic patients in Swedish primary health care and in the general population: comparison between 1992 and 1995. *Qual Life Res*, 1998, 7:751-760.

[73] Wandell P. E. Quality of life of patients with diabetes mellitus: an overview of research in primary health care in Nordic countries. *Scand J Primary Health Care*, 2005, 23:68-74.

[74] Collins M. M. et al. Quality of life and Quality of care in patients with diabetes experiencing different models of care. *Diabetes Care*, 2009, 32(4):603-605.

[75] Colquitt J. L. et al. Clinical and cost-effectiveness of continuous subcutaneous insulin infusion for diabetes. *Health Technol Assess.*, 2004, 8:1–171.

[76] Bradley C., Speight J. Patient perceptions of diabetes and diabetes therapy: assessing quality of life. *Diabetes Metab Res Rev.*, 2002, 18(Suppl 3):S64–S69.

[77] Hoogma R. P. et al. Comparison of the effects of continuous subcutaneous insulin infusion (CSII) and NPH-based multiple daily insulin injections (MDI) on glycemic control and quality of life: results of the 5-nations trial. *Diabet Med*, 2005, 23:141–147.

[78] Tsui E. et al. Intensive insulin therapy with insulin lispro: a randomized trial of continuous subcutaneous insulin infusion versus multiple daily insulin injection. *Diabetes Care*, 2001, 24:1722–1727.

[79] Davis R. E. et al. Impact of hypoglycemia on quality of life and productivity in Type 1 and Type 2 diabetes. *Curr Med Res Opin.*, 2005, 21:1477–1483.

[80] Linkeschova R. et al. Less severe hypoglycemia, better metabolic control, and improved quality of life in Type 1 diabetes mellitus with continuous subcutaneous insulin infusion (CSII) therapy; an observational study of 100 consecutive patients followed for a mean of 2 years. *Diabet Med.*, 2002, 19:746–751.

[81] Nicolucci A. et al. Quality of life and treatment satisfaction in adults with type 1 diabetes: a comparison between continuous subcutaneous insulin infusion and multiple daily injections. *Diab Med*, 2008, 25:213-220.

[82] WHO: *Adherence to Long-Term Therapies*. Evidence for Action. 2003, World Health Organization, 3-4.

[83] Gerber K. E., Nehemkis A. M. *Compliance: the dilemma of the chronically ill.* New York, USA: Springer Publishing Company, Inc.; 1986.

[84] Ajzen I., Fishbein M. Attitudes and the attitude-behavior relation: Reasoned and automatic processes. *Eur Rev Soc Psychol.*, 2000, 11:1-34.

[85] Feinstein A. R. On white-coat effects and the electronic monitoring of compliance. *Arch Intern Med.*, 1990, 150:1377-1378.
[86] UK Prospective Diabetes Study (UKPDS) Group: Intensive blood-glucose control with sulphonylureas or insulin compared with conventional treatment and risk of complications in patients with type 2 diabetes (ukpds 33). *Lancet*, 1998, 352:837-853.
[87] UK Prospective Diabetes Study (UKPDS) Group: Effect of intensive blood-glucose control with metformin on complications in overweight patients with type 2 diabetes (ukpds 34). *Lancet*, 1998, 352:854-865.
[88] Bergman U., Wilholm B. E. Drug-related problems causing admission to a medical clinic. *Eur J Clin Pharmacol.*, 1981, 20:193-200.
[89] Cramer J. A. A systematic review of adherence with medications for diabetes. *Diabetes Care*, 2004, 27(5):1218-1224.
[90] Testa M. A., Simonson D. C. Health economic benefits and quality of life during improved glycemic control in patients with type 2 diabetes mellitus: a randomized, controlled, double-blind trial. *JAMA*, 1998, 280(17):1490-1496.
[91] Pibernik-Okanovi M. Psychometric properties of the World Health Organization quality of life questionnaire (WHOQOL-100) in diabetic patients in Croatia. *Diabetes Res Clin Pract.*, 2001, 51(2):133-143.
[92] Lau C. Y. et al. Association between glycemic control and quality of life in diabetes mellitus. *J Postgrad Med.*, 2004, 50(3):189-93.
[93] Weinberger M. et al. The relationship between glycemic control and health-related quality of life in patients with noninsulin-dependent diabetes mellitus. *Med Care*, 1994, 32(12):1173-1181.
[94] Goddijn P. P. et al. Longitudinal study on glycemic control and quality of life in patients with Type 2 diabetes mellitus referred for intensified control. *Diab Med.*, v. 16(1), p. 23-30, 1999.
[95] Kleefstra N. et al. Cross- sectional relationship between glycemic control, hyperglycemic symptoms and quality of life in type 2 diabetes (ZODIAC-2). *Neth J Med.*, 2005, 63(6):251-221.
[96] Pitale S, Kernan-Schroeder D, Emanuele N, Sawin C, Sacks J, Abraira C: Health-related quality of life in the VA Feasibility Study on glycemic control and complications in type 2 diabetes mellitus. *J Diabetes Complications,* 2005, 19(4):207-211.
[97] Pippalla R. S. et al. Interrelationships of quality of life, compliance, clinical outcomes and life satisfaction: a cross-sectional study on hypertensive geriatrics. *J Clin Pharmacy Ther.*, 1997, 22(5):357–369.

[98] Sung J. C. et al. Factors affecting patient compliance with anti-hyperlipidemic medications in an HMO population. *Am J Manag Care*, 1998, 4(10):1421-1430.

[99] Holzemer W. L. et al. Predictors of self-reported adherence in persons living with HIV disease. *AIDS Patient Care STDS*, 1999, 13(3):185-197.

[100] Billups S. J. et al. The relationship between dug therapy noncompliance and patient characteristics, health-related quality of life, and health care costs. *Pharmacother.*, 2000, 20(8):941-949.

[101] Cote I. et al. Is adherence to drug treatment correlated with health-related quality of life? *Qual Life Res.*, 2003, 12(6):621-633.

[102] Duran-Varela B. R. et al. Pharmacological therapy compliance in diabetes. *Salud Publica Mex.*, 2001, 43(3):233-236.

[103] Hernandez-Ronquillo L. et al. Factors associated with therapy noncompliance in type-2 diabetes patients. *Salud Publica Mex.*, 2003, 45(3):191-197.

[104] Martínez Y. V. et al. Quality of life associated with treatment adherence in patients with type 2 diabetes: a cross-sectional study. *BMC Health Services Res*, 2008, 8:164-175.

[105] Gregg E. et al. Diabetes and physical disability among older U.S. adults. *Diabetes Care*, 2000, 23:1272–1277.

[106] Jacobson A. M. et al. The evaluation of two measures of quality of life in patients with type 1 and type 2 diabetes. *Diabetes Care*, 1994, 17:267–274.

[107] G'Afvels C. et al. Living with diabetes: relationship to gender, duration and complications: a survey in northern Sweden. *Diabet Med.*, 1993, 10:768–773.

[108] López R. K. et al: The CALVIDIA Group. Perceived mental health at the start of dialysis as a predictor of morbidity and mortality in patients with end-stage renal disease (CALVIDIA study). *Nephrol Dial Transplant.*, 2004, 19:2347–2353.

[109] McEwen L. N. et al. Are health related quality of life and self-rated health associated with mortality? Insight from Translating Research Into Action for Diabetes (TRIAD). *Prim Care Diab.*, 2009, 3:37–42.

[110] Kleefstra N. et al. Prediction of mortality in Type 2 diabetes from health related quality of life (ZODIAC-4). *Diabetes Care*, 2008, 31:932–933.

[111] Tibblin G et al. Quality of life as an outcome variable and a risk factor for total mortality and cardiovascular disease: a study of men born in 1913. *J Hypertens.*, 1993, 11:S81–S86.

[112] Brown S. E. S. et al. Perceptions of quality-of-life effects of treatments for diabetes mellitus in vulnerable and non-vulnerable older patients. *JAGS*, 2008, 56:1183-1190.

[113] Van der Zee K. I. et al. The psychometric properties of the SF-36-item Short Form Health Survey in a Dutch population. *Tijdschrift voor Sociale Gezondheidszorg*, 1994, 4:183–191.

[114] Landman G. W. D. et al. Health-related quality of life and mortality in a general and elderly population of patients with type 2 diabetes (ZODIAC-18). *Diabetes Care*, 2010, 33:2378-2382.

In: Quality of Life in Endocrine Diseases ISBN: 978-1-63463-911-8
Editor: Erika Cesar de Oliveira Naliato © 2015 Nova Science Publishers, Inc.

Chapter 9

Obesity and Quality of Life

Renata A. Mendes and Erika C. O. Naliato *
Center of Studies Ricardo A T Castilho of the Teresópolis
Medical Association, Brazil

Abbreviations

AC	Abdominal Circumference
BAROS system	Bariatric Analysis and Reporting Outcome System
BMI	Body Mass Index
IDF	International Diabetes Federation
IWQOL-Lite questionnaire	Impact of Weight on Quality of Life – Short form
NCEP	National Cholesterol Education Program
PedsQL questionnaire	Pediatric Quality of Life Inventory
QoL	Quality of life
WHR	Waist–Hip Ratio

* Correspondence to: erikanaliato@uol.com.br.

Introduction

Obesity is defined as the excess of adipose tissue in the organism, and has multifactorial causes, involving genetic and environmental factors. A family-linked inheritance is perceived in which children of obese parents have a higher risk of being obese themselves [1].

Obesity is a chronic disease considered one of the most relevant public health problems to the extent that it constitutes an important risk factor for the development of various diseases, such as Diabetes Mellitus, hypertension, dyslipidemia, hyperuricemia, coronary artery disease, cerebrovascular accident, osteo-arthritis, sleep apnea, respiratory problems, biliary lithiasis, endometrium, breast, prostate, and colon cancers [1, 2, 3].

Over the last years, obesity has been considered a real epidemic with the emergence of new cases in developed and developing countries [1, 2, 3].

Weight excess affects approximately one-third of the adult population, and its incidence has been increasing in the last decades. There is a higher prevalence of obesity in women, especially those coming from poorer socio-economic classes in developing countries, while, in the developed ones, the incidence in men and women is similar. In both genders, the highest levels occur in people aged between 45 and 64 [1, 3].

Besides that, obesity is associated with an increase of morbidity and mortality due to cardiovascular diseases [4]. Between the non-cardiovascular complications of obesity, non-alcoholic steatohepatitis draws the attention, for which the most effective treatment seems to be gradual weight loss [4].

Despite the high accuracy of the complementary methods of diagnosis of obesity, their elevated costs and operational complexity raise difficulties in using them in the day-by-day clinical practice. Considering this, the anthropometric measurements represented by Body Mass Index (BMI), Waist–Hip Ratio (WHR), and Abdominal Circumference (AC), function as a sensible and efficient way of estimating volume and fat distribution; therefore, they should be used in the everyday clinical practice [2, 3].

Using the BMI as reference, individuals who present a value equal or higher than 30 kg/m^2 are considered obese. Considering the WHR of the general population, individuals are considered to have central obesity when they present WHR higher than 0.9 in the feminine gender and 1.0 in the masculine. In relation to the AC, in accordance to the NCEP (National Cholesterol Education Program) criteria, it is possible to consider the diagnosis of abdominal obesity from 102 cm in men and 88 cm in women, and there is a substantially increased risk of obesity-associated metabolic complications in people with these measures [2, 3].

The International Diabetes Federation (IDF) recommends other cut-off values in relation to abdominal circumference for the rise in risk of metabolic complications: 80 cm for the feminine gender and 94 cm for the masculine [2, 3]. Other factors may influence the prevalence of obesity. In a study developed by Kac et al. (2001) [5], there was a higher prevalence of abdominal obesity (AC superior to 80 cm) in women with two or more children and over 35 years old. Nowadays, there are a variety of effective options for the treatment of overweight and obese patients, including food diet, physical activity, behaviour therapy, pharmacotherapy, surgery, and combinations of these techniques [2, 6]. Many factors must be considered at the moment of the choice of treatment. Characteristics such as AC, BMI, presence of risk factors, and the patient's motivation to lose weight may affect the commitment to the therapy [6]. The motivation may be estimated by the previous history of weight loss in earlier treatments, whether it was well succeeded or not. The support of family and friends to the patient's attempt to lose weight, the accessibility of time to proceed with the treatment, the social-economic conditions, and the patient's cognitive capacity may affect the commitment to the treatment and prevent relapses [2].

The initial objective of the therapy is a 10% reduction of the weight in a six-month period. After this interval, the weight loss rhythm usually declines due to a reduction on the basal caloric expenditure [6]. Studies demonstrated that the weight reduction lowers blood pressure, the levels of triglycerides, total cholesterol and the LDL fraction, insulin resistance, as well as cardiovascular risk to diseases [2].

The strategies for weight loss and its maintenance are:

Dietary therapy and physical activity suitable to each individual in addition to the cessation of tobacco smoking are recommended [2, 6]. Despite weight gain being a usual collateral effect after the cessation of smoking, this immediate weight gain does not exclude the possibility of a long-term weight reduction [2].

The dietary therapy associated with the multidisciplinary therapy (nutritional education, regular physical activity, change of eating behaviour, and hypocaloric diet) in patients with obesity was globally linked to an average reduction of 11 cm in the abdominal circumference, reduction of the prevalence of metabolic syndrome in 50%, and reduction of hypertension in all participants, with a remarkable improvement in the quality of life (QoL) [7, 8].

Drugs are recommended to aid in the treatment of patients with: (1) BMI values higher or equal to 30 kg/m² or (2) BMI values higher or equal to 27 kg/m² with presence of risk factors, comorbidities, or obesity complications [2, 6]. Pharmacological treatment must be obligatorily associated with appropriate diet and adequate physical activity [2].

The following comorbidities or complications are considered important symptoms for the association of pharmacological therapy: hypertension, dyslipidemia, coronary heart disease, Diabetes Mellitus type 2, and sleep apnea [2, 6]. The continual evaluation by the physician is necessary to ensure the effectiveness and security of the treatment [2].

The bariatric surgery must be conducted in patients with BMI higher or equal to 40 kg/m² or in those with BMI higher or equal to 35 kg/m² associated to the presence of comorbidities [2, 6].

Quality of Life in Obesity

In comparison to smoking and drinking, obesity is related to a worse QoL [9]. Conversely, weight loss is associated with an improvement in the QoL of obese people. The loss of 10% or more of the original weight in the period of one year is linked to the improvement in all the dimensions of the IWQOL-Lite questionnaire (Impact of Weight on Quality of Life – Short form), which evaluates physical function, self-esteem, and aspects such as public and work discomfort [10]. In a study conducted in 2011, Vasiljevic et al. [10] verified only one exception when it comes to the improvement in the QoL after weight loss: sexual activity.

The presence of comorbidities may deepen the QoL deficit in obese people. An example of this is approached in the study of Olczyk et al. (2010) [11]. According to the authors, there is additional worsening in the QoL in obese patients with growth hormone deficiency.

QoL Evaluation Instruments Specific for Obese People

The PedsQL questionnaire (Pediatric Quality of Life Inventory) is a generic version for children may be used in the evaluation of the QoL related to the health of obese children [12].

One of the QoL questionnaires specific for the obese is the IWQOL Lite [13]. In a study carried out in Brazilians, the Brazilian version of the IWQOL Lite questionnaire was presented as the first specific instrument validated in Brazil to evaluate the QoL in obesity. This version of the questionnaire may be used both in epidemiological studies and in activities of health assistance in order to evaluate the treatment therapies adopted for obese individuals [13].

Another questionnaire used in the evaluation of the QoL of the obese is the Laval Questionnaire. This questionnaire constitutes a valid measurement of health, is especially related to the QoL in patients with morbid obesity, and is sensitive to the changes induced by the treatment [14].

The BAROS system (Bariatric Analysis and Reporting Outcome System) uses a scoring table (in which the maximum score corresponds to 9) to evaluate the weight loss, the complications, the improvement in health conditions, and the QoL in the patients during the postoperative of bariatric surgery. This scoring table has confirmed itself to be valid and trustworthy. BAROS scores above 7 are considered excellent [15].

Quality of Life in Obese Patients

Zabelina et al. (2009) [16] investigated the association between age, weight, and QoL. The impact of weight was evaluated through the IWQOL-Lite questionnaire. The age increase stimulated the influence of the weight in the QoL related to physical function, sexual life, and work. Despite that, the age increase was associated with lower impairment of self-esteem and anguish than with weight gain. In this study, women's scores in all IWQOL-Lite domains were significantly lower, denoting a higher harm to their QoL than to men's.

Oliva-Moreno & Gil-Lacruz (2011) [17] analysed the relationship between weight and QoL and their results revealed a link between weight excess and a decrease of QoL. The study revealed that the negative effect of weight excess was felt more acutely in the dimensions of life related to mobility and pain/discomfort, also indicating important differences between genders and age groups. Women and elderly people were more likely to suffer the negative consequences of weight excess. These data confirm those obtained by White et al. (2004) [18] which indicated that Caucasian women presented a higher impairment of QoL.

Men with abdominal circumference equal or higher than 102 cm, including those non-obese (BMI inferior to 30 kg/m^2), have QoL deterioration, with symptoms of impairment of physical, psychological, and sexual functions [19]. The promotion of health aiming at the improvement of the QoL must focus on the prevention of obesity and central fat accumulation [19].

Psychopathologic disorders are the most relevant factors associated with the impairment of QoL of poor obese patients, affecting not only the psychological domain in itself, but also the physical, in the majority of cases, independent of the severity of the obesity. Interventions of psychological and psychiatric nature are fundamental for a global treatment of obesity, to improve the results of treatment, and reduce relapse [20]. According to Barajas-Gutiérrez et al. (1998) [21], the profile of obese patients with the worst QoL is of a woman aged over 50 with low educational level and affected by psychiatric disease.

Quality of Life in Obese Patients Treated by Gastroplasty

According to Padwal et al. (2010) [22], the bariatric surgery is presently the most efficient treatment available to obese patients; it is associated with the reduction of morbidity and mortality and improvement of QoL. This kind of treatment significantly reduces the patient's weight, lessens the necessity of medical care and health expenses [22, 23].

Laparoscopic Roux-en-Y gastric bypass obtained good results for weight loss and its maintenance for a period of seven years. The majority of patients have improvement in QoL and all comorbidities evaluated, which leads to good up to excellent results in five years in 97% of the evaluated patients according to the BAROS score [24].

QoL was evaluated before and on the years 1 and 5 of postoperative after gastrectomy for morbid obesity in a study conducted in Finland. The Moorehead-Ardelt questionnaire was used for the evaluation. The treatment of morbid obesity by gastrectomy provided an improvement in QoL in all the domains maintained for 5 years. Despite that, after the surgery, the QoL index related to age and sex was still worse than the one found in the general population [25].

Quality of Life in Obese Children and Adolescents

In children, obesity can be associated to psychosocial problems including social marginalization, low self-esteem, and damaged QoL; therefore interventions in the lifestyle are recommended including adequate food diet, physical activity and, in selected cases, the performance of bariatric surgery [26]. Bariatric surgery is superior to the isolated changes in lifestyle in the treatment of morbid obesity in adolescents [27]. Obese children present inferior QoL in relation to eutrophic children, with significant differences in the physical, emotional, social, psychosocial domains and QoL in general [12, 28]. In comparison with healthy adolescents, those overweight or obese have QoL inferior in all the domains [29, 30]. Girls may present even greater effect of overweight and obesity in QoL [29].

Quality of Life in Obese Elderly Patients

Obesity is a disease with high prevalence in elderly people, which contributes to the appearance of chronic diseases and functional incapacity, being related to precocious mortality. The prevalence of obesity increases with age leading to a significant physical deficiency as well as to a higher prevalence of metabolic syndrome and to the detriment of QoL. As a result, the control and proper management of obesity in this group of patients become important with the intent to reduce precocious morbidity and mortality [31].

Conclusion

Presently, obesity is considered one of the most relevant public health problems to the extent that it constitutes a risk factor for various diseases such as hypertension, Diabetes Mellitus, dyslipidemia, coronary artery disease, hyperuricemia, cerebrovascular accident, osteoarthritis, sleep apnea, respiratory problems, biliary lithiasis, endometrium, breast, prostate, and colon cancers, all which can be prevented by weight loss [1, 2, 3]. The loss of 10% or more of the original weight in the period of one year is associated with an improvement of the QoL [5]. And this improvement occurs in many subpopulations of obese people - obese men and women, gastrectomized patients, children, adolescents, and the elderly [21, 22, 30]. Taking this into consideration, it is important to promote population awareness aiming at the change of Western habits linked to regular physical activity, healthy eating, drug and/or surgical treatments in selected cases for weight loss.

References

[1] Gofin, J et al. The prevalence of obesity and its changes over time in middle-aged and elderly men and women in Jerusalem. *Int J Obes.*, 1996; 20:260-266.

[2] Department of Veterans Affairs, Department of Defence (VA/DoD). VA/DoD clinical practice guideline for screening and management of overweight and obesity. National Collaborating Centre for Primary Care/National Institute for Health and Clinical Excellence (NCCPC/NICE). Obesity: the prevention, identification, assessment and management of overweight and obesity in adults and children. 2006; 1-84.

[3] Obesity: preventing and managing the global epidemic. Report of a WHO Consultation on Obesity, Geneva, 3-5 June 1997. Geneva, World Health Organization; 1998. WHO document WHO/NUT/NCD/98.1. Accessed via http://whqlibdoc.who.int/hq/1998/WHO_NUT_NCD_98.1_ (p1-158).pdf and http://whqlibdoc.who.int/hq/1998/WHO_NUT_NCD_98.1_(p159-276).pdf in April/2011.

[4] Manton N. D. et al. Non-alcoholic steatohepatitis in children and adolescents. *Med J Aust.*, 2000, 173 (9):476-479.

[5] Kac G., Velásquez-Meléndez G., Coelho M. A. S. C. Fatores associados à obesidade abdominal em mulheres em idade reprodutiva. *Rev Saúde Pública,* 2001, 35(1):46-45.

[6] Considine, RV & Caro, JF. Obesity: The problem and its management. DeGroot L; Jameson J (ed). *Endocrinology*. 6th ed. Philadelphia, USA: W. B. Saunders Company: 2010; 1:555-565.

[7] Arrebola E. et al. Evaluation of a lifestyle modification program for treatment of overweight and nonmorbid obesity in primary healthcare and its influence on health-related quality of life. *Nutr Clin Pract.,* 2011, 26:316-321.

[8] Bischoff S. C. et al. Multicenter evaluation of an interdisciplinary 52-week weight loss program for obesity with regard to body weight,

comorbidities and quality of life-a prospective study. *Int J Obes.*, 2012, 36(4):614-624.
[9] Klijs B., Mackenbach J. P., Kunst A. E. Obesity, smoking, alcohol consumption and years lived with disability: a Sullivan life table approach. *BMC Public Health,* 2011, 11:378.
[10] Vasiljevic N., Ralevic S, Kolotkin RL, Marinkovic J, Jorga J. The Relationship Between Weight Loss and Health-related Quality of Life in a Serbian Population. *Eur Eat Disord Rev.*, 2012, 20(2):162-168.
[11] Olczyk J., Kokoszko A., Lewiński A., Karbownik-Lewińska M. Quality of life and exercise capacity in obesity and growth hormone deficiency. *Neuro Endocrinol Lett.*, 2010, 31:700-707.
[12] Poeta L. S. et al. Qualidade de vida relacionada a saúde de crianças obesas. *Rev Assoc Med Bras.*, 2010, 56(2):168-172.
[13] Mariano M. H. et al. Psychometric evaluation of a Brazilian version of the impact of weight on quality of life. *Eur Eat Disord Rev.*, 2010, 18(1):58–66.
[14] Therrien F., Marceau P., Turgeon N., Biron S., Richard D., Lacasse Y. et al. The laval Questionnaire. A new instrument to measure quality of life in morbid obesity. *Health Qual Life Outcomes*, 2011, 9(1):66.
[15] Al Harakeh A. B., Larson C. J., Mathiason M. A., Kallies K. J., Kothari S. N. BAROS results in 700 patients after laparoscopic Roux-en-Y gastric bypass with subset analysis of age, gender, and initial body mass index. *Surg Obes Relat Dis.*, 2011, 7:94-98.
[16] Zabelina D. L., Erickson A. L., Kolotkin R. L., Crosby R. D. The effect of age on weight-related quality of life in overweight and obese individuals. *Obesity,* 2009, 17(7):1410-1413.
[17] Oliva–Moreno J. & Gil- Lacruz A . Body weight and health-related quality of life in Catalonia, Spain. *Eur J Health Econ.*, 2013, 14(1):95-105.
[18] White M. A., O'Neil P. M., Kolotkin R. L., Byrne T. K. Gender, Race, and Obesity-Related Quality of Life at Extreme Levels of Obesity. *Obes Res.*, 2004, 12:949-955.
[19] Han T. S., Tajar A., O'Neill T. W., Jiang M., Bartfai G., Boonen S., et al. Impaired quality of life and sexual function in overweight and obese men: the European Male Ageing Study. *Eur J Endocrinol.*, 2011, 164:1003-1011.
[20] Mannucci E. Petroni M. L., Villanova N., Rotella C. M., Apolone G., Marchesini G., QUOVADIS Study Group. Clinical and psychological

correlates of health- related quality of life in obese patients. *Health Qual Life Outcomes,* 2010, 8:90.

[21] Barajas-Gutiérrez M. A., Robledo Martín E., Tomás García N., Sanz Cuesta T., García Martín P., Cerrada Somolinos I. Quality of life in relation to health and obesity in a primary care Center. *Rev Esp Salud Publica*, 1998, 72:221-231.

[22] Padwal R. S., Majumdar S. R., Klarenbach S., Birch D. W., Karmali S., McCargar L., et al. The Alberta population- based prospective evaluation of the quality of life outcomes and economic impact of bariatric surgery (APPLES) study: background, design and rationale. *BMC Health Services Res.*, 2010, 10:28.

[23] Mäklin S., Malmivaara A., Linna M., Victorzon M., Koivukangas V., Sintonen H. et al. Cost-utility of bariatric surgery for morbid obesity in Finland. *Br J Surg.*, 2011, 98(10):1422-1429.

[24] Suter M., Ralea S., Millo P., Allé J. L. Laparoscopic Roux-en-Y gastric bypass: significant long-term weight loss, improvement of obesity-related comorbidities and quality of life. *Ann Surg.*, 2011, 254:267-273.

[25] Helmiö M., Salminen P., Sintonen H., Ovaska J., Victorzon M. A 5-Year Prospective Quality of Life Analysis Following Laparoscopic Adjustable Gastric Banding for Morbid Obesity. *Obes Surg.*, 2011, 21(10):1585-1591.

[26] Canoy D., Bundred, P. Obesity in children. *Clin Evid (online)*, 2011, pii: 0325.

[27] Bondada S., Jen H. C., Deugarte D. A. Outcomes of bariatric surgery in adolescents. *Curr Opin Pediatr.*, 2011, 23(5):552-556.

[28] Ottova V., Erhart M., Rajmil L., Dettenborn-Betz L., Ravens-Sieberer U. Overweight and its impact on the health-related quality of life in children and adolescents: results from the European KIDSCREEN survey. *Qual Life Res.*, 2012, 21(1):59-69.

[29] Al-Akour N. A., Khader Y. S., Khassawneh M. Y., Bawadi H. Health-related quality of life of adolescents with overweight or obesity in the north of Jordan. *Child Care Health Dev.*, 2012, 38(2):237-243.

[30] Riazi A., Shakoor S., Dundas I., Eiser C., McKenzie S. A. Health-related quality of life in a clinical sample of obese children and adolescents. *Health Qual Life Outcomes,* 2010, 8:134.

[31] Donini L. M. et al. Obesity in the elderly. *Ann Ig.*, 2011, 22:499-511.

Acknowledgments

The authors would like to thank our families for their everlasting love, support and encouragement and our patients for allowing us to be part of their lives.

To my mentors, Alice Violante and Annamaria Colao, for sharing their wisdom.

Index

R

S

T

W